Dear David

Thank you for all your concern & wise counsel.

God bless

With love

Hazel

Learning to be the patient:

a doctor's cancer journey

(with spiritual and ethical reflections)

Hazel J Butland

authorHOUSE®

AuthorHouse™
1663 Liberty Drive, Suite 200
Bloomington, IN 47403
www.authorhouse.com
Phone: 1-800-839-8640

© *2008 Hazel Butland. All rights reserved.*

No part of this book may be reproduced, stored in a retrieval system, or transmitted by any means without the written permission of the author.

First published by AuthorHouse 7/10/2008

ISBN: 978-1-4343-9696-9 (sc)

Printed in the United States of America
Bloomington, Indiana

This book is printed on acid-free paper.

This book is dedicated to the memory of

Lorna Blissett

27 June 1964 – 2 December 2007

My own cancer journey would have been so much harder

without her friendship support and experience

My journey begins

On Sunday 1 October 2006 my daughter Rachel phoned me from Manchester where she had just started a very intensive postgraduate music course at the Royal Northern College of Music. She's a cellist. I pretended everything was normal at this end. She was getting herself very worked up because she felt she could not play the piano adequately. She needed to practise! She was living with pianists but there was no piano. I suggested a keyboard but she dismissed this suggestion. She didn't want to practise at the Royal Northern because she was embarrassed about her ability.

She was inconsolable. Of course, we all get upset at times but this was ridiculous. In the end, I suggested she took her music with her to the school, where she was teaching the following day, to see if she could use one of their pianos, but she wasn't happy. I couldn't drive up to Manchester and buy her a keyboard, just like that. This was ridiculous! Anyway, I had other things on my mind.

The following evening she phoned again. She was better! She said everything had changed, it was all right now! She had returned to the house after teaching practice; she walked into their shared living room and noticed the furniture had been moved round. Sitting in the corner was a piano. It had just arrived. She had no idea it was coming! The landlady needed somewhere to store it!

It seemed that God was shouting to us all: 'Stop worrying, I will provide! I will care for all your needs.'

I didn't tell her about the breast lump. What would have been the point of worrying her unnecessarily?

The following evening I was diagnosed with breast cancer.

As I look back, this incident constantly amazes me. The timing was perfect: a little incident, but so precious. Something to remember when things are getting on top of us!

Introduction

At the beginning of October 2006, at the age of fifty, I was diagnosed with breast cancer.

Overnight my life was turned upside-down. I was working part-time as a general practitioner in the community, and at the local hospice, and as a forensic medical examiner (police surgeon) for the Thames Valley police. I am a wife, and a mother, and as a Christian, also fortunate to be a member of a caring Christian community. Suddenly, my life had changed: I was no longer the one who juggled numerous jobs, and provided care; I was the one who needed help and support. I was still a doctor, but suddenly I was also a patient, with a long journey ahead of me.

Shortly after I was told I had breast cancer I started a journal. Initially, it was mostly reflective, but I began a far more systematic journal later in my journey. At Christmas I bought a laptop and that made it so much easier. Little did I know how invaluable that would be. By February I was suffering from severe ankle swelling, which made sitting at a desk very uncomfortable. I could work on my laptop whilst reclining on the settee, or in bed.

Keeping a journal was new to me – after all with at least three jobs I didn't have time, but the idea came to me within days. Although I hadn't kept a journal, I had discovered the value of writing. I had just completed a philosophy and medical ethics dissertation. This had involved reflecting on the ethical management of cancer patients, so I resolved to write reflectively on topics, as they came up. I had learnt the therapeutic benefit of writing reflectively whilst writing up case histories for my dissertation. Sitting down at the computer, and reflecting constructively on a patient's story, can be so rewarding. Examining feelings of anger, frustration, inadequacy, sadness or even joy can be such a benefit for future patients.

At the start of my journey, I didn't know what would happen; I didn't know how events would unfold. As things progressed, I realised that emotional, physical and spiritual problems should also be recorded, as they took place. The nature of the journal evolved and changed. I became more dependant on it as a coping mechanism.

I have, therefore, added some narrative to the reflections at the beginning of my journey.

I have placed the more reflective passages in italics to distinguish these from the more straightforward narrative. Some of the reflections are spiritual; I hope these will help my friends. Some of the reflections are ethical, or more medical; I hope these will interest my colleagues, and others working in the field.

Reflection: when did my journey begin?

I stood by the canal at Broughton, on the outskirts of Aylesbury, in reflective mood. I looked back towards Aylesbury town, and ahead towards Marsworth, where our branch of the canal joins the main Grand Union Canal. The canal doesn't start at Broughton, it starts in Aylesbury, and like the canal's journey, my cancer journey didn't start when I was diagnosed, it had started sometime earlier. I was expecting bad news, although I was uncertain what was going to happen.

As a family we were being prepared for a crisis, each in our own way. As Christians we believe in a loving heavenly Father who cares for us, and provides for all our needs, but he doesn't promise a life without troubles.

For my husband, I think the journey began when he decided to get rid of his old Vauxhall Astra. He really wanted to buy a more environmentally friendly car. At the end of July we test drove a Toyota Prius, which fully satisfied his need for a 'green' car. I was happy too, my husband had a new 'toy', and it was far more comfortable for a passenger, than the Astra. As he usually cycles to work, he only uses his car for longer journeys. When we bought it, we had no idea how much travelling around the UK we would be doing, later in the year – after all our planned holiday was a trip to China in October.

For Marian, I believe her journey began when she decided to turn down the opportunity to tour with a Christian theatre company, for six months, choosing instead to remain in London. As an actor, this was a difficult decision, but at the time she had no idea how much both her mother, and her grandmother, would need her cheerful company over the time she would otherwise have been away.

For Rachel, the situation was rather different. She had just started a very intensive music teaching course. However, she had planned to have a 'gap' year after completing her degree in Sheffield in June, before applying for the postgraduate teaching course. The situation changed when she discovered September 2006 was going to be the last intake for that particular course. She frantically applied when she was also completing her degree. If she had had a gap year, she might have been travelling abroad when I discovered I had breast cancer.

Unfortunately, whilst Rachel had been taking her finals in Sheffield in May/June 2006, the mother of one of the girls in her string quartet died of breast cancer. This naturally had a profound effect on her reaction to my diagnosis, four months later.

For me, the most significant event occurred just before Easter 2006, although I had been attending a one-year postgraduate course, in philosophy and medical ethics, since September 2005. Just before Easter, my friend Lorna came to see me at the surgery. She was not only a friend, but also a patient and a colleague. She is an experienced palliative care nurse, and like me she worked at the hospice. A few weeks earlier we had been discussing the essay she was doing on 'death and dying' in palliative care. When Lorna came to see me, we were shocked to find that she had a large abdominal mass which turned out to be ovarian cancer. Before her diagnosis was confirmed, Lorna and I had another chat. We chatted about my decision to write a medical ethics dissertation on the use of the 'four principles' approach to biomedical ethics, in cancer and palliative care. We both knew the principles, first described by Beauchamp and Childress, that can be used to guide ethical decision making: respect for autonomy (or free will, freedom of choice), beneficence (doing the best for the patient), non-maleficence (not doing harm), and justice (fairness, appropriate use of resources). In our discussion, Lorna was a great advocate for autonomy, and the importance of allowing patients to make their own decisions. I argued that in cancer care it is often impossible for patients to make appropriate decisions, and they needed gentle guidance to help them make rational decisions. Doing what is best for the patient (beneficence), being such an important aim of hospice care. When we were discussing this, I had no idea Lorna would become one of the cases in my dissertation, and, of course, I had absolutely no idea how important her support, experience and friendship would become when I too was diagnosed with cancer, six months later.

Lorna, in fact, reinforced my own argument, and acknowledged the weakness of her own, when she came back to me, after she had seen the gynaecologist. Should she have surgery? Was it worth it? What should she do? Was the effort of going through chemotherapy going to be worthwhile? Her mind was in turmoil, she needed guidance. She wanted to know what was best.

This reinforced my argument, that although we should respect the autonomy of a cancer patient, they may well need help to make rational decisions.

My dissertation was completed at the beginning of September. Exactly a month later, I discovered I had breast cancer, and faced similar turmoil to Lorna, although I was offered the possibility of cure. Even so, I really didn't want to have to make decisions. I'm a GP but

I wasn't thinking rationally. I knew I wasn't. At least I had argued that clearly in my dissertation! As far as I was concerned it was totally appropriate to allow the consultants to make the decisions. They are the experts, anyway. If I had felt I needed to be more involved in the decisions, I would have needed to spend time looking up the information on the internet. I was not ready to do that; in fact it was not until I knew I needed a mastectomy, six week later, that I felt able to look up anything about breast cancer on the internet.

I am so grateful that I was able to reflect on this, talk this through with Lorna, and write it up before I knew I was ill.

There are two other recurring themes from my dissertation.

The first is the necessity to listen carefully to a patient, to ensure we really do understand their needs. This is particularly important in palliative care, when patients often struggle to express their needs. It takes time, so it is important to make it clear you have plenty of time to listen. I always try to sit down at the bedside during my hospice ward rounds. Listening involves watching, observing the patient's behaviour, as well as weighing up the words spoken by the patient.

The second important topic was the significance of casuistry in the ethical management of palliative care patients. Casuistry is the examination and study of individual cases. Learning from an individual's experience may have a profound effect on subsequent ethical decisions. It is a very natural way to work. We should learn from people's stories. We thrive on stories! I learnt a great deal from Lorna, and it has helped me. I hope my story will help others too, but we must remember that we are all different; we react to suffering in different ways. I must be careful, in the future, not to assume that others will have exactly the same thoughts and experiences as I have had. Even so, it is important to me, to believe that my experience may be helpful to others, both colleagues and patients. It's helpful, along my journey, to feel others might be helped through my suffering.

Journal

Monday 25 September

We came back from a wonderful party yesterday evening. We went up to Stockport for the weekend, to celebrate the twenty-fifth wedding anniversary of Alison and Chris, who both trained with me in Sheffield in the 1970s. We celebrated with a barn dance on Saturday night. I hadn't been to a barn dance for years. It was great fun, and we met so many people we hadn't seen for a long time. Rachel, our daughter, came too.

Earlier in September our younger daughter, just turned 21, had moved to Manchester after graduating in music from the University of Sheffield, to start an intensive PGCE (postgraduate certificate in education) at the Royal Northern College of Music (RNCM) in Manchester.

I also took the opportunity to look at the Royal Northern and a bit of Manchester. Yesterday, we worshipped with Rachel at Ivy Cottage, the church she has just joined. It was a very special service. The worship leader was amazing. She has a fantastic gift: singing out prophetically, whilst improvising on her guitar; it was beautiful. The preaching by Debra Green was also excellent. I feel sure Rachel has found the right place to worship, and grow in her Christian faith.

Unfortunately, one thing is bothering me. After the barn dance we went back to our hotel, and whilst lying in bed, I am increasingly aware of pain in my right breast.

I can't make up my mind what's going on. Both my breasts are very lumpy, and since starting on HRT (hormone replacement therapy) almost exactly three years ago, my breasts have enlarged, and become more difficult to examine. There seems, however, to be a more clearly defined lump at the side, in the upper, outer quadrant. I know I don't check my breasts very often; perhaps a case of 'practise what I preach rather than what I do', but I am sure I would have noticed this, if it had been there for a while. Anyway, why does it hurt so much? As a GP I often reassure patients that if it hurts, it's generally not cancer. Is that right? I'm only taking very low-dose HRT, but I could stop it for a few days, and see what happens.

Wednesday 27 September

The tender area in my right breast seems less obvious today, and there is a similar lumpy area in the left breast, but not quite as obvious, and not painful. I'll see what it's like tomorrow.

Thursday 28 September

I had to go down to High Wycombe this evening, to discuss the rota with the other police surgeons in the area. I found it really hard to concentrate; the pain in my breast is getting worse. Every time my right arm presses against it, it is horrible, and the pain is like 'toothache' all the time. I know I had a cyst in that breast in the past, but I couldn't feel it; maybe it has suddenly got bigger. I have got to get something done about it; I can't stand the pain much longer.

Friday 29 September

The *Independent* arrived this morning with the entire front page covered with the latest breast cancer statistics, introducing 'Breast Cancer Awareness' month. Trust me to find a breast lump at the beginning of 'Breast Cancer Awareness' month!

Immediately after my morning shower, I decided to ring for an appointment to see my GP. It's rather alarming to think I needed an article all over the front of the *Independent* to give me enough courage to phone for an appointment.

I sat on the side of my bed, in my underwear, and picked up the phone. It was nearly 8.30 a.m. I got through, the line wasn't engaged, and I spoke to the receptionist. I asked for an urgent appointment, so she asked me what the problem was. I wondered if my receptionists would have asked that, but I didn't mind. I'm glad I was honest. As soon as I said 'breast lump', she told me the GP registrar's 8.40 a.m. appointment had just cancelled. Could I make it in time? I said 'yes' and 'thank you', thinking, 'little does she know what I am wearing at present!' I dressed very fast, leapt into the car, and drove to the surgery.

As I was sitting in the waiting room, I was wondering if the young doctor would really want to see me. She has just spent three months working at the hospice with me. It can be so hard seeing a colleague, especially one so much older.

She called me in, and we examined the lump together. I told her I would make my own appointment to see Alan, the breast surgeon, as I have private health insurance through my husband's work.

When she examined the breast, we agreed the lump had a smooth outline, and was about 3 cm in diameter. We both agree it could well be a cyst.

I phoned the Chiltern Hospital as soon as I got home. I'm going to see the surgeon next Tuesday evening. At least that's sorted, but my breast still hurts.

I've got a very busy weekend coming up; how can I cope with going up to London tomorrow, with the pain in my breast?

I can't believe how silly I've been! When patients come to me complaining of headache or joint pain, and haven't taken any painkillers, I'm amazed at their foolishness, but that's exactly what I've been doing. I don't need to put up with the pain; I can at least see if it settles with ibuprofen! I suppose I didn't want to cover up the symptoms, before getting it seen, and that's what the patients think too.

Saturday 30 September

What a day!

The pain in my breast has settled considerably with anti-inflammatory medication, so I did go to London. Today was the start of the new academic year at the Society of Apothecaries, for the history of medicine course, and philosophy of medicine course (ethics and philosophy of healthcare). I have just completed the philosophy of medicine course; I loved it! I love learning new things and reflecting on new ideas. I wish the course had been longer. Anyway, I have decided to continue studying. Helen, the hospice consultant, and I have agreed to start the history course together, although she will miss some lectures this term. We have decided to do the course over two years.

We travelled up on the train together. I decided to warn her about my appointment, trying to reassure her and myself, that it would be a false alarm. We laughed! She was going to be off work for a while, and we had no specialist registrar, and now I couldn't guarantee being around either! I am sure they will manage without us.

I love Apothecaries' Hall. It is a wonderful building tucked away in Black Friars Lane. There is a life-sized painting of a cousin of my father, hanging in the room where I sat my philosophy diploma and the diploma in medical jurisprudence!

After the lecture we had a reception. I then had a chat with Don, the philosophy of medicine tutor. I'm not sure if he has marked my dissertation yet – it's another month before we hear if we have passed. I'd love to know! We talked about unethical management practices. He challenged me to write up my traumatic experience in what appeared to be a very dysfunctional general practice. I agreed it might be constructive; after all, it might well help me to come to terms with it. But I am so busy. When on earth will I find time to sit down, and type up the scribbled notes, from all those years ago? I know they are in the house somewhere, but have I got the courage to read them again? Mightn't it just bring back memories that would be better kept buried?

(I eventually wrote up an account of my time at this practice which I considered very dysfunctional during March 2007. Details and reflections are under the heading 'The play within the play'. To conceal its identity I have just called it the 'dysfunctional practice.')

I had arranged to meet Marian, my 23-year-old daughter later in the afternoon. She is an actor, living in London, and earning enough to pay the rent by teaching dance and doing promotional work. I hope she gets some more paid acting work soon! She has a strong Christian faith, and worships at Kensington Temple, although she sometimes goes to Hillsong instead with her housemates.

During our meal together at a restaurant, I told her about the lump in my breast. I find Marian so easy to talk to, and easy to confide in. Although she looks like a teenager, and that's her acting age, I often find her very wise and mature in her understanding. I told her that I had an appointment on Tuesday evening, and she said she would pray for me, and phone after the appointment.

I have decided not to mention it to Rachel. She's still adjusting to her new course, and she may not need to know. I don't want her worrying more than necessary.

October 2006

Sunday 1 October

We had such a difficult phone call from Rachel today; she was so worried about where she would be able to practise the piano. She certainly wasn't in the right frame of mind to tell her about my breast lump. Anyway, it may not be necessary at all.

Monday 2 October

It was such a very long day at work today, and I didn't concentrate very well. I told my partners Kate and Joe about my appointment. Kate was very reassuring. After all, the lump is painful; therefore it might not be cancer.

But I'm worried. Since I started ibuprofen the lump has changed in its nature. It's less swollen, but no longer smooth in outline. It is now an irregular mass. I am sure it is malignant. I'm sure I have breast cancer.

We received another call from Rachel this evening. What an amazing solution to all her stress. A piano has turned up in her house! I hope, after all that fuss, she makes the most of it!

Tuesday 3 October

I work at the hospice on Tuesday mornings. I see the in-patients and try to spend time in the day hospice. I love to eat my lunch with the day-patients. It is good to get to know the patients when they are reasonably well. They may become in-patients in the future. It gives me time to listen. Sometimes conversations can be so special.

Giving patients time is so important. Recently, I have been examining my practices, in the light of my philosophy and ethics dissertation, concerning ethical decision-making in cancer and palliative care. I have started doing my ward round carrying round a chair to sit on. I want patients to realise I have time for them.

I also want to attend Holy Communion with the patients more often. I love the simple service and gain from the support of David the hospice chaplain too.

I didn't concentrate very well at work today, but Helen, my consultant, was very caring. The lump seems huge. How could I have failed to feel it before? But both breasts feel much less lumpy in general, apart from the mass, so it's easier to feel.

This afternoon I was asked to attend Aylesbury police station to take forensic samples from a prisoner. I got quite stressed as I realised I was running out of time, and might not get to my outpatient appointment in time. I'm afraid I was a bit rude to the custody sergeant, when he started asking me further questions. I told him I had to go. I would be on call from 7 p.m., but not before.

At the Chiltern Hospital I was called in to see Alan, the surgeon. I was worried that I was wasting his time, and didn't want to appear to be neurotic. He was very kind. He thought he would just have to aspirate a cyst for me. When he started to examine my breast, his body language changed. It was clear he was worried. He was concerned and caring but said little; he didn't need to, apart from saying that we had better get on with a mammogram, scan and biopsy immediately.

As I waited for my mammogram I found myself praying. I was not praying for help, or that the problem would go away; I was saying 'thank you.' Thank you that I was being taken seriously, and I wasn't wasting everyone's time. Before performing the mammogram, the radiographer asked me where the lump was. I looked down at my breast and pointed. I said: 'It's really rather obvious, you can see it.' As I said this I started to tell myself off. How could I possibly have failed to detect such an obvious lump, sooner? What must Alan think? I'm a GP, and I allowed my own breast lump to get this big! What sort of GP am I? Maybe just a very busy one, who doesn't have time to look after herself.

After the mammogram, I was ushered in to see the radiologist, for the ultrasound scan and biopsy. As soon as she placed the ultrasound probe on my right breast, over the lump, I could see that the architecture of the breast was abnormal. She measured a 3 cm mass.

The enormity of the situation started to dawn on me, as I lay there. She asked me what Alan had said to me. I told her he had said very little, but his silence and concern had told me everything. She explained the procedure for the biopsy to me and, after numbing the area, she sampled the mass.

Alan was waiting for the result of the scan. Before he spoke to the radiologist, he asked me what she had said. I told him it wasn't good news. We then had a further chat about management. There was no pretence, no saying 'we need to wait a week for the biopsy result.' The situation was clear, and we needed an immediate management plan.

He suggested neo-adjuvant chemotherapy to reduce the size of the mass, and make the surgery less invasive.

His idea is for me to have six cycles of chemotherapy, and then a lumpectomy, followed by radiotherapy. He was very kind, but when he asked me what I thought about the plan, I had no idea. How could I make any decisions? I was dazed; it was all so unreal, was this really happening to me? OK, I can help my patients make reasoned decisions, but this was different. It's me we were talking about! I told Alan that I wanted him to make the decisions. That was one thing I was completely clear about. I'd just spent weeks writing up my dissertation on ethical decision-making in cancer and palliative care. I'd discussed and reflected on autonomous decision-making at diagnosis with my friend, patient and nurse colleague, Lorna. Six months ago she had been adamant that our palliative care patients should make their own choices, until she discovered she had cancer. Suddenly things changed, and she couldn't think rationally; she asked me what she should do, what would be best. That's exactly what I wanted too; the specialist to make the decisions for me.

We agreed to his plan, but I would need to be referred to an oncologist for the chemotherapy so he asked me which oncologist I wanted to see. Even that was a difficult question! I said I would like to see the Oxford based oncologist Amanda, and he said he would organise it, but I should phone her. The sooner I started chemotherapy the better.

I went back to my car. I was in complete turmoil. The police needed me to see a prisoner in High Wycombe police station, but I needed to start telling people the bad news. But first, I needed to come to terms with it myself. I drove the eight miles to High

Wycombe, planning what to do. I knew I would have to drive the sixteen miles back to Aylesbury, as well, but I couldn't possibly carry on all night with the on-call, driving backwards and forwards between Aylesbury and Wycombe. It would be totally irresponsible. When I reached Wycombe custody, I told the jailer that I needed to make some phone calls, before seeing the prisoner. I phoned Pedro, one of my colleagues, and he immediately agreed to take over the on-call for the rest of the night. That was a great relief.

I needed to start telling people. I hadn't even told my husband, Nick. Tuesday evening is chess club. I couldn't phone him until he got home. I waited and phoned him from the doctor's room in custody. I said I would be driving back soon, and asked him to have a glass of wine ready, because I needed it.

Helen, the hospice consultant phoned. She was so kind and told me I really shouldn't be at work!

Then Marian phoned. She had been thinking and praying about me. She was spending the evening with some close Christian friends. I was so relieved she was with friends to support her, one of them a junior doctor. I told her I did have breast cancer. She started to cry; somehow I had to comfort her. I hate telling bad news over the phone. I wanted to hug her and I couldn't. I could hear her friends chatting in the background; she said they were in another room. I tried to encourage her to go and talk to her friends, but she didn't want to. I had to think quickly. I told her to phone home, and talk to her dad. At least they could support each other. That helped and comforted me whilst I saw the prisoner.

The prisoner was a long-term alcoholic and drug addict and needed medication to help him overnight. Whilst chatting to him my phone rang again. It was Joe, my senior partner at the practice. In front of the prisoner, I told Joe that I did have cancer, and asked him to tell Kate, our other partner. When I stopped talking on the phone, the prisoner was looking at me with amazing compassion. He was so sorry and said his problems were trivial compared to mine.

I promised to sort out his medication, and as he left the room, he wished me well. This level of concern and compassion from a prisoner was very special.

I drove home. I sat down on the settee, with Nick, with a glass of wine in my hand, and wept. I was mentally and physically exhausted.

Wednesday 4 October

Nick took the morning off work. There was so much to do, so much to come to terms with; so much had changed.

I phoned my Mum.

I hate telling people over the phone, but I have no choice: I want to be the one to tell them. So many people still think cancer means they will soon be attending a funeral. I want to be the one to reassure them, to talk of the hope of a cure, not to be 'all doom and gloom', to show them I can still laugh.

Nick drove me to work. Kate greeted me with concern and compassion written all over her face. We said little, just hugged. Nick and I then both went upstairs to talk to Rachel, my practice manager. She was shocked, but we agreed that we would call all the staff together at the end of morning surgery, and I would tell them. They hugged me. I really felt loved. In the midst of suffering, it was very special.

We cancelled my afternoon surgery, and after lunch I was going to have a sleep, when I thought, 'I must phone the GP registrar who

I saw last week.' I didn't want her to find out by reading it in an impersonal letter, or – worse still – not to find out at all. She was shocked and surprised, but I assured her the lump had changed in its feel after she had seen me. She had not made a mistake in thinking it was benign, after all, so had I. She promised to let Andy, my actual GP know.

At teatime the phone rang again; it was Andy. I am so fortunate to have such a caring GP. He is also the GP in charge of the day-to-day running of our local cancer and chemotherapy unit. He has invited me to go and see it and talk through the treatment tomorrow, after I have finished at the hospice.

I still need to speak to my daughter Rachel. She will have been teaching in schools all day, and she is still not answering her mobile. I have had to leave a voicemail message to get her to phone me back. That's the last thing I wanted to do, but I must speak to her today. I know she will be upset.

Thursday 5 October
Learning to be the patient

Rachel eventually phoned back at 9 p.m. last night. She had just finished lectures – what an intensive course. I gave her the news. It was a harrowing experience.

I need time to reflect on it. There is only one sensible thing to do. The most constructive way for me to deal with my frustrations, sorrows, anger and distress is to write it up as a reflection, perhaps for teaching ethics in the future. I hope that writing up my reflections will help me cope with my illness. If I keep a journal of my journey, at least I will have something to show for my extended sick leave. I can submit it next July for my annual GP appraisal. I'm 'learning to be the patient'.

Andy showed me round the chemotherapy unit. He showed me the scalp-cooling machines. He explained that they were designed to cool the scalp, to try to limit hair loss. He said I could choose to wear it during my chemo, if I wanted. Otherwise, my hair is likely to fall out after three to four weeks. I said I would think about it. I then sat and watched whilst Andy wrote up my chemotherapy, sending the order to the pharmacy so I could start my chemo next Tuesday.

Suddenly, the reality of my situation was brought home to me. Next week, I would really be having chemotherapy. It wasn't a dream. It wasn't a game. It wasn't an educational tutorial: I was the patient, and I was going to start a therapeutic journey that could be very difficult.

Andy assured me that breast tumours can respond well to neo-adjuvant chemotherapy, that they can shrink away to almost nothing. Of course, I will still need to have the area excised after I have finished the treatment, but I will keep most of my breast.

He told me that the plan is for me to attend the unit for intravenous chemotherapy once every three weeks, for six cycles. They will give me treatment to stop me feeling sick, but I must be very careful during the second week of the three-week cycle, because my white cell count will be very low. I will become neutropenic (low neutrophil count). It is the neutrophil white cells in the blood that protect against bacterial infection. I need to be on my guard against tonsillitis, cystitis and food poisoning, for example. Bacterial infection in this situation can be fatal. Of course I already knew this but it alarmed me, and again brought home to me the situation I'm in.

Friday 6 October.

This morning Nick took me over to the Churchill Hospital in Oxford to meet Amanda, my oncologist. She was really supportive. She agreed with the plan, but as yet we haven't received the histology report. We agreed that I would commence the chemotherapy FEC (5-fluorouracil, epirubicin and cyclophosphamide) on Tuesday, provided the histology report confirms the diagnosis. That is highly likely.

We talked about the fact Nick and I are due to fly to China for a fortnight's holiday, in ten days' time. Poor Nick's so looking forward to going but we agreed that it would be foolish. If I definitely have cancer, we need to cancel the holiday.

Saturday 7 October

Breaking bad news

I had always maintained the importance of face-to-face contact when telling anyone bad news. I had even been quite dogmatic about this on the philosophy of medicine course, criticising a colleague for arguing how much easier it is to tell people bad news over the phone, rather than speaking to them face to face. It may be easier for the doctor not to have to deal with the emotional response close at hand, but how can you comfort someone over the phone? How can you gauge the reaction and ensure the recipient of bad news is composed enough to drive, or continue working? Only by having eye contact can non-verbal communication be accurately assessed. Listening to the reaction of the recipient of bad news is far more than just hearing the response and the tears over the phone. Listening includes close observation.

This is fine in theory, but how could I tell my family that I had been diagnosed with breast cancer face to face, when they were living miles away? It was so much easier to tell colleagues and friends, as I could speak to them directly and hug them – I've never been hugged so much in my life!

I had to rethink my approach to communicating bad news. A landline would be better than a mobile phone. As my mother pointed out, concerning my sister in California: what if she's driving when I contact her?

If phoning is impossible, then email or letter-writing would be better than text-messaging. This is far too informal, and again, the recipient could be anywhere at the time. Any communication in writing is far poorer than direct communication. Over the phone at least it is possible to comfort and assess the person's reaction to some extent, but the consolation of a hug or just touching the person is far better.

Ideally, I wanted to speak to members of my family when there was at least a possibility that someone would be with them, but how can you guarantee this when you are phoning them? My mother lives on her own, but at least she is in a flat, with others around.

It was easier to convey the bad news to those to whom I had mentioned that I had found a breast lump, and who knew I had an appointment with the consultant. For me it was important to try to anticipate the way the recipient of my news would react before telling them. This, of course, varied, depending on whether the person was a female relative, a daughter, my husband, a work colleague, a friend or a patient.

For my medical colleagues, I anticipated concern and compassion, but of course there were also significant implications for their workload. I managed to tell most of the staff at the surgery face to face. It was fantastic to realise how much they care, but also to realise how much I am valued by my staff, and particularly by my practice manager.

Of course, I even had to tell my husband over the phone, as he didn't attend the initial consultation with me, and because I had not anticipated getting the diagnosis immediately. At least he knew I was seeing the consultant, and we had time together, and some wine later in the evening. It also gave me the opportunity I needed to cry.

I am glad I had had a meal with my daughter Marian in London three days earlier, and had told her about the appointment. At the time I wasn't sure whether this was sensible, as at that stage I still thought it would be a benign cyst, and would worry her unnecessarily. She was clearly anxious, and was thinking about and praying for me. When she phoned me on my mobile phone whilst I was at the police station, I had to break the news to her. She immediately burst into tears – conveying to me how much she loves me – but how could I console her? Fortunately, she was having a meal with three close Christian friends, one of whom is a junior doctor. This, at least made it easier for me to feel she would be supported. I also told her to phone home and chat to her father – support for both of them. She had also already arranged to visit her grandma (my mother) two days later, so I knew they would support each other.

Marian's love and support turned out to be even more important when communicating the news to Rachel, her younger sister. As Rachel had only just commenced her PGCE in Manchester, and was finding some of the work very stressful, I had chosen not to worry her, so she didn't know I had found a breast lump. As I knew she would be in school all day, I planned to phone her early on Wednesday evening. I would have to phone her on her mobile, and I wanted her to be with friends, when I rang. Unfortunately, I had to leave a voicemail message the first time I tried.

She eventually phoned back at 9 p.m. I asked her if she was with friends. She replied that she was entirely on her own at the Royal

Northern College of Music, and had just finished lectures. I had to tell her, but I knew it would be difficult. She sobbed her heart out, and became quite angry. 'I hate it' was her cry, but this was not surprising. Her experience of breast cancer, so far, has been supporting two of her closest friends – one at school, and one just four months ago at university – when both their mothers died of breast cancer. It made me realise how significant case histories are. My experience of breast cancer is so completely different from my daughter's. Marian hasn't had the same sort of experience. In fact, the mother of her closest friend, who has had breast cancer in recent years, is well and almost certainly cured.

Perhaps it was a good thing that Rachel was on her own at the RNCM, as the acoustic is so immense, and her sobs echoed throughout the building. She was also angry with me for not warning her, and telling colleagues before her. This was hard to manage, and I had to try to calm and reassure her. All she wanted to do was come home to give me a hug. I hoped she would be going back to her house immediately, but she said she was planning to go and practise after the call.

I was so grateful I had arranged with Marian, beforehand, to phone her immediately after I had finished on the phone, so she could speak to her sister to support her. She phoned her sister, and then spoke to her the next morning as well. I received a very reassuring text message from Marian the following morning.

The following day, I spent time trying to persuade Rachel not to get on a train and come rushing home at the weekend; I tried to persuade her to go and visit our friends in Stockport instead. However, apparently she had started to cry in one of her tutorials, and the course organiser was very supportive, saying that if she needed to go home, that was fine. Amazingly, Rachel's friend Alex, in the second year of the course and whose family live near us, heard about the situation and immediately offered her a lift home for the weekend in her car. She said that she had woken up the weekend before and thought, 'Rachel will need a lift home next weekend.' The Lord knew that, but at that time none of us did!

It was lovely to be able to give Rachel a big hug when I saw her, and we had twenty-four hours with Marian at home as well. The girls filled the house with singing and laughter, as they role-played each other's dance and music lessons. This transformed the atmosphere of the house, and I had a weekend to cherish: a special gift.

Marian and Rachel went to church together and met up with friends. They were supported by the close fellowship that was a great comfort for me.

Alex and Rachel also had the opportunity to celebrate Hannah's birthday – their mutual friend – who lives on our estate. This was important as Hannah survived acute myeloid leukaemia, and Hannah's mother Joy reminded Rachel that she had had treatment for breast cancer fifteen years ago.

Rachel showed me how much she loved me in all this; it was very special.

Trying to let my younger sister, Christine, know what was happening was even more problematic as I was giving her the news over the phone and all I had was a mobile phone number.

I discussed with my mother what to do, as Christine lives and works in California. Her great anxiety was that she might be driving when I phoned. The first time I tried, I got her voicemail but was unable to leave a message as I didn't understand the instructions. This meant she would know she had had a missed call from the UK. My concern, then, was she would assume it was 'bad news' about our mother. I sent her an email (which she didn't open until after my second, successful phone call) to make it clear I wanted to talk about me. I phoned her *again the following day, and timed it accurately for her lunch hour in the physiotherapy department.*

Poor Christine had had a dreadful week and this was the last straw. She burst into tears, sobbing over the phone because she couldn't give me a hug. After trying to comfort her, I asked her whether she was working in the afternoon, to which she replied that she was about to sit a two-hour physics exam. I felt awful, but I had had no idea. What a terrible situation to be in; I had tried so hard to anticipate this sort of thing, but hadn't anticipated this scenario. Fortunately, she still passed the exam!

Finally, I wanted to break the news personally to a friend whose wife had died some years ago, and I guessed she had died of cancer. I didn't want him to hear via the grapevine, and I certainly didn't want to tell him via email. I realised it was important to find out more about his wife, before I told him my story. The last thing I wanted to do was tell him I had breast cancer, 'which the doctors are aiming to cure with treatment', if his wife had died in similar circumstances. Sadly, his wife had died of cancer, but not breast cancer. It was good to talk, and allow him to talk, but I am glad I approached the situation sensitively.

Sunday 8 October

After the girls left, I decided I needed to spend some time quietly, reflecting and praying. I could have gone to the evening service, but I chose to be alone. I drove to Broughton to walk beside the canal.

Monday 9 October

Today was my last full day working at the surgery. I have annual leave anyway, so I will decide how much work I can continue to do once I've discovered how I cope with chemotherapy.

I had to phone Alan's secretary during morning surgery, to see if she could get hold of my histology report. I can't start chemo without confirming I have breast cancer, but I don't want any delay, and I'm meant to be starting tomorrow.

At the end of morning surgery the phone went, and it was Alan himself at the other end. It was so good to speak to him personally. He said the histology confirms breast cancer, but that I have a lobular tumour, not the more usual ductal carcinoma. He explained that 10 to 15 per cent of breast tumours are lobular tumours, and these are the ones that are much more difficult to detect. They don't show up on mammograms in the same way as ductal tumours do, and can be difficult to detect on ultrasound scanning. He also said they are difficult to feel. He said that that explains why it got to this size before I felt it.

What a relief! Suddenly a huge weight has been lifted off my shoulders.

I thanked him for phoning, but especially for saying that. Maybe he himself had wondered how I had allowed the lump to get to this size, but now he has reassured me that he understands.

Well, at least I know I will definitely be starting chemotherapy tomorrow.

Tuesday 10 October

I was due in the chemotherapy unit at 10 a.m. today. I popped into the hospice first for some moral support and some toast.

It was going to be a long day. I eventually decided to try the scalp cooler, to see if I could prevent my hair falling out. That meant having the refrigerator-like headgear on for an hour prior to chemo, and ninety minutes afterwards, to try to constrict my scalp blood vessels sufficiently to prevent the chemo reaching those hair follicles. It can go to other parts of my body, and, most importantly, to the tumour, and any area of tumour spread. One lady who's having the same treatment as me still has wonderfully long hair.

It was my daughter Rachel's wise remark that convinced me to try scalp cooling. She said: 'Try it the first time to see how you get on; this is a learning experience that you can pass on to your patients!'

The cooler certainly made me feel very cold, and rather faint. Fortunately, I started to feel faint before I was given the chemo, so I knew it wasn't that!

The chemo nurse was very good, but as I sat watching her, as she gave me the injections of chemotherapy, it seemed unreal. She was injecting the drugs into a drip attached to an arm. Was that really my arm? Were those drugs really going into me? Surely I was just a doctor observing what was going on; how could I possibly be the patient as well?

The side-effects have convinced me otherwise. I have been given quite a cocktail of medication to counter the sickness, including the strong steroid dexamethasone, which I need to take for the next three days.

Friday 13 October

Well, I went into work at the hospice yesterday, even though I had my first chemotherapy on Tuesday. I didn't know how I would feel, but I was determined to try. I wanted to talk to people about it. I knew I would benefit from the support.

Recently, I have been thinking about what is important in my work, especially in day hospice and my role there. It is very easy to pop down to day hospice to eat, but without spending time with the patients. Sitting down to have lunch with them gives time to listen, time for conversation to develop, and time for questions, but only if I am committed to being there. Occasionally, really important topics are raised, but not often; it requires time, patience and perseverance.

I resolved to spend more time with the patients over lunch.

Yesterday I sat down in day hospice with a few patients and staff, to chat with them before lunch. I wasn't sure if I would be too tired to have my lunch with them. I started to tell the patients about an occasion, some years ago, when a day patient asked me during lunch, 'Do you think we are terminally ill?'; I was surprised to find myself answering, 'No! You are living with cancer, not dying of it.'

After telling the story, I explained to the patients that now I too am living with cancer, and had had my first dose of chemotherapy on Tuesday. One of the ladies said she had seen me there.

Later, when I had completed my morning's work, I was feeling light-headed and very hungry. I needed to take my medication, but I had to take it 'with food', and the side-effects of the steroid dexamethasone were making me feel very hungry. It was an excellent time. The experience of sharing with the patients was amazing. I didn't need an excuse to be there, and their support was wonderful.

I'm not just the doctor who assesses the patients any longer; I'm one of them too.

Monday 16 October
Plymouth: time to reflect

Today we should have been flying off to China. Poor Nick, he really wanted to go, but how could we? We would have been cruising down the Yangtze at exactly the time when I would have been most susceptible to infection. I would have been so anxious, I wouldn't have enjoyed it. Anyway I'm tired and breathless; I couldn't have kept up with the group.

Instead we are in Plymouth and I have plenty of time to reflect. It is great to read some spiritual reflections by others. I'm new to this type of work. I am only just discovering the quality of the literature the Catholic Church has produced in a reflective style.

Henri J.M. Nouwen, in his book of the same title, asks the question: 'Can you drink the cup?' reflecting on the words of Jesus, in Matt. 20: 20–23, to James and John. The cup is a cup of suffering, but ultimately also a cup of joy.

'Just living life is not enough. We must know what we are living. A life that is not reflected upon isn't worth living... Half of living is reflecting on what is being lived. Is it worth it? Is it good? Is it bad?... Holding the cup of life means looking critically at what we are living... Holding the cup of life is a hard discipline' (pp 26–7).

My friend Shirley lent me this book. I had asked her to lend me Nouwen's reflections on The Return of the Prodigal Son, *but she lent me this one instead! I had never heard of the Catholic priest's reflections until Laurence, our vicar, read a section from* The Return of the Prodigal Son, *at an evening service, last month. The timing was perfect* and Shirley's apparent mistake was no mistake at all. This short book, *Can you Drink the Cup?*, has become such a blessing to me since my diagnosis. Can I drink the cup of suffering that lies before me; will it become a cup of joy?

Spiritual reflection: my walk beside the canal last Sunday

On the Sunday after I discovered I had breast cancer, I couldn't go to church in the evening – I didn't feel like singing. I didn't want noise, I wanted solitude. I needed time to reflect. Time to reflect on the cup (of suffering) I had been given, and to reflect on the path that had been mapped out for me over the next year.

I wanted time to reflect on God's amazing provision for me.

Not then to ask: 'Why me?' After all, the obvious answer to that is: 'Why not?' Ultimately, I wanted to reflect on the way I had been prepared to take hold of, accept, and drink the cup given to me to carry.

By the time I was ready to seek my place of solitude, the sun had set, but there was still light in the sky. I chose the canal at Broughton and started walking east, away from Aylesbury. Skeins of geese flew across the canal, to the meadow on the other side. A few ducks were enjoying an evening dip, and a solitary robin sang its melancholy autumnal song as a bat flew round and round above the tow path.

As I was beginning to walk back, I became aware of a white glow in the sky on the horizon. It took a few seconds to realise that, in fact, it was the full moon rising; a huge cream-coloured disc, slowly emerging and illuminating a single bush, from behind, silhouetting it, and highlighting it against the darkening sky. My mind was drawn to the moment when Moses spotted the bush in the desert that was burning but never consumed by fire. This was when God spoke to Moses, and revealed

His name to him, 'YHWH' (Yahweh), translated 'I AM' or, 'He who IS/The one who IS' (Exod. 3:14), the God who is, and always has been, without beginning or end.

The moon waxes and wanes, it comes and goes, but God is constantly present, watching over us.

Slowly, the moon rose higher until it was high enough for me to see its reflection in the still waters of the canal. As I looked at the straight canal stretching out into the darkness I thought about the journey I was starting out on and realised it had started a while before I knew about the diagnosis. The canal doesn't start at Broughton; it begins (or ends) in Aylesbury. Likewise, my journey didn't start here. Planning for the journey started as I began to focus on my dissertation, and began in earnest at Easter when Lorna was diagnosed with ovarian cancer.

I reflected that the path was laid out before me and I had to follow it, but God was watching over me, illuminating my path and leading me beside still waters. The beginning of psalm 23 was very much on my mind.

The Lord is my shepherd; I shall not want.
He makes me lie down in green pastures.
He leads me beside still waters.
He restores my soul.
He leads me in paths of righteousness for his name's sake.
Even though I walk through the valley of the shadow of death,
I will fear no evil;
For thou art with me;
Thy rod and thy staff, they comfort me.
(Revised standard version)

The sheep in the field, illuminated by the light of the moon, were lying down in green pastures and even though I was walking through the valley of the shadow of death, I had nothing to fear.

I hadn't wanted to go to church for the evening service; I knew I wouldn't cope. However well-meaning they might have been, I wasn't ready to be prayed for in front of the whole congregation, and I didn't want inappropriate prayer. Yes, I wanted prayer for healing, but I wanted meaningful prayer. Whatever happened, I would still need chemotherapy, surgery and radiotherapy. Anything less would have been against expert medical advice based on the medical findings.

The more I reflect on this special moment beside the canal the more precious it becomes; after all, the moon waxes and wanes and often rises long before, or after, sunset.

I had to be standing beside the canal at the exact time the moon rose. The moon had to rise after dark to stand out so clearly. Only a full moon could have drawn my attention to the bush so specifically. If the moon had risen any later I would have gone home as there would not have been sufficient light to continue my walk. There were clouds in the sky but not obscuring the moon.

I believe my presence there at that moment was stage-managed by our wonderful creator God, who cares for the individual and desires a personal relationship with us, whatever the circumstances.

Tuesday 17 October

Did I know I was going to suffer? That sounds like a ridiculous question, but it is very profound as well.

Can I drink the cup of suffering? Was I prepared to go through suffering again was a question that I had been asking myself for several months.

Why?

I was very aware that spiritually and emotionally I was very happy, just like I was during the time when our children were little, immediately before I was plunged into a very traumatic situation within the dysfunctional practice. At that time, and again this year, I was very satisfied with my work and feeling I was achieving good results. Spiritually, I was well supported by strong church home group then and again, during the last year, this has been the case.

Recently, although I found the challenge of studying philosophy and medical ethics very rewarding, it has made me reflect again on what happened at that surgery. The focus on the ethics of healthcare has reminded me of my time at this unethical, dysfunctional practice. Maybe, during the long months ahead between chemo sessions I will have time to write it up after all.

Wednesday 18 October

It's just over a week now since I had my chemotherapy. I must be so careful to avoid infection. I'm washing all fruit and salad and we are picking our restaurants carefully! I've got my electronic thermometer with me and I am taking my temperature twice daily but it seems to be low rather than high! I'm very tired. I'm having a two-hour sleep most afternoons and I can't walk very far. I'm getting breathless very quickly. We park and I can walk downhill to a pub or restaurant but Nick goes to get the car on the way back. It's hard to believe how little I can manage.

For the last few days I had been taking a sleeping tablet to help me get to sleep. I had been struggling to sleep following chemotherapy as the stimulant effects of dexamethasone had been keeping me awake. Last night, I decided to try sleeping without a sleeping tablet and was reasonably successful apart from the vivid dreams.

What are dreams? In this case it was certainly an expression of my suppressed fears.

I had gone to sleep after watching two television programmes. The first was *Holby City* but with the specific theme of assisted suicide – a woman going to Switzerland to die. The second programme was a documentary about the first lady to have a partial face transplant. It took place in France. She had an amazingly good result – but what a risk, and what about the future?

My nightmare was about the horrors of a recurrence of breast cancer on the chest wall. This dream highlighted for me my greatest fear. It's what happened to a patient I recently looked after in practice. I woke up and reminded myself that she had rejected conventional medicine. I resolved, once again, to follow all the advice of the experts.

Over the last few days I have become more reflective. It's hard to reflect when 'high' on dexamethasone, but my mood has slowly become more normal. I have started thinking about the future. I have been telling people that 'I have a 70 per cent chance of cure – and that is without prayer!' That's fine, but when my mood is low I think about the 30 per cent.

Even if I have a long remission I will always live with uncertainty – I know that.

I have again been reading from Henri Nouwen's reflections in *Can you Drink the Cup?* It has helped me to think about what is important. He, as a catholic priest, described the huge difference between standing officiating in front of the congregation and sitting down around a table and sharing communion as part of the community. Isn't that what it is like to sit and eat a meal with the patients, or sit down to talk to in-patients on the ward round, rather than standing dominating the situation?

Maybe I ought to have a cup of coffee with the in-patients more often!

Whilst we were standing looking at the sea Nick said to me: 'When I die, I want my ashes scattered in Plymouth Sound. Where do you want your ashes scattered?' I paused for a moment reading between the lines. Poor Nick clearly felt he needed to introduce the subject of my death, but had wondered how to do it. I was impressed by his courage and thought quickly. I replied, 'Hermaness!' So he replied, 'In which case I'm dying first!' Well, I have chosen my favourite place. I mean it; I would love my ashes to be scattered at Hermaness, the most northerly point on Unst, the most northerly of the Shetland Isles. Yes, OK, it's a two-mile walk over peat bog to get there, and it is usually blowing a gale at the high cliff edge, but the puffins and gannets are wonderful!

Friday 20 October
<u>Our wedding anniversary – twenty-seven years of marriage!</u>

Of course we should have been in China but instead we travelled back from Plymouth. Nick isn't the only Plymothian in our church.

We are very fortunate to have friends who have a house there to rent and was available 'at the last minute'. We were surrounded by love and compassion whilst we were there. It was great to see Nick's uncle Bob and aunt Christine again, as well as Auntie Win who, at the age of ninety+ is healthier than I am at present! She has wonderful memories of Plymouth between the wars. She proudly showed us the articles in the *Plymouth Herald* recently written about her and her brothers.

Tomorrow we are spending the day at home but on Sunday we are going to visit my older sister, Jenny, and brother-in-law, Chris, in Keighley, West Yorkshire. We haven't stayed with them for years! They have a lovely house high up on one side of the valley.

When we arrived home there was a note from a florist saying they had failed to deliver some flowers whilst we were away. I rang them immediately and they are going to deliver them tomorrow!

Saturday 21 October.

The flower arrangement has arrived; it is magnificent! It's from my Auntie Gladwys in Rochdale. It's great, the flowers don't need to be transferred to a vase and the packaging will protect them. That means we can take the arrangement with us on our travels. Everyone can enjoy them!

Tuesday 24 October

We had a lovely walk along the canal near my sister's yesterday. I can walk further now, provided it's reasonably flat!

This morning there was a lovely sunrise. There was a mist in the valley but you could see the hills beyond. I tried to photograph it but didn't really capture the beauty. A watercolour painting would be better but that's not one of my gifts!

We are travelling to the Lake District today. We managed to get a midweek deal at the country hotel for three days, even though it's half-term! It's great because it is also Rachel's half-term holiday so she is travelling up from Manchester to join us, and Marian is coming up from London too. It's years since we had a family holiday. OK, Nick and I aren't in China but we are having time with our family instead. I feel the girls need to see that their mum is still alive and smiling.

As we were saying goodbye to Jenny some redwings were eating the red berries in her rowan tree. These are the first redwings I have seen this autumn. They are lovely birds. Winter will be here soon!

Wednesday 25 October

On our way over to the Lake District we stopped and had a walk up to Malham Cove. What a spectacular place! We spotted a young lad with a telescope. He was extremely excited. There was a peregrine falcon sitting on a dead branch. He was trying to photograph it. I had a go too. I have a good zoom on my camera but I have noticed I have developed a tremor since starting chemo. I really needed a tripod, but resting the camera on Nick's head worked quite well!

I discovered a new trick as well. It wasn't easy to point out the peregrine to other walkers, but once I had taken its photo I could show it to them on the screen. They could then immediately spot the location and see it for themselves. Digital photography has many advantages!

The hotel is wonderfully situated overlooking Lake Windermere and the food is fantastic! Auntie Gladwys's flower arrangement looks great in our hotel bedroom. It's still travelling with us. We've arranged to visit her on our way home. I hope it will still be looking good.

It was a beautifully calm day so the girls went kayaking and had a brilliant time. Nick and I went for a walk. I climbed a hill; I made it! I am recovering well now. It's good to think I will have a few days feeling well before my next chemo on Tuesday.

Thursday 26 October

I phoned Rachel, my practice manager, today. I have decided I can manage morning surgery twice a week. I can't work afternoons; I need to sleep! I will be working Monday and Friday mornings at the surgery and Tuesday and Thursday mornings at the hospice.

After our walk yesterday I noticed something odd. My scalp was hurting; in fact it's very tender. I think my hair's starting to fall out. It doesn't look as if the scalp cooler has worked for me. It's falling out sooner than I had expected. I wonder if the wig I ordered will be there when we get home!

Friday 27 October

Marian travelled back to London overnight – she's had two auditions today for pantomime; I hope she gets one of them!

We travelled home via Manchester. We were going to drop Rachel off at the station but realised it would be just as easy to take her back to her house. We then went to visit my Auntie Gladwys. She has been a widow for some time, but with the help of excellent professional carers and her family, she looks after her two teenage grandsons, James and Daniel. Both boys live with Duchenne muscular dystrophy. James is eighteen now and needs constant help with his breathing but Daniel still zooms around in his wheelchair.

It was a very special time, and she saw the flower arrangement too!

Tuesday 31 October

I had my second lot of chemo today. I have decided not to wear the scalp cooler any more – after all, my hair is falling out anyway. It's pretty horrible; the hair gets everywhere. Handfuls come out when I shower but overnight it's all in the bed as well. I'm going to have the rest cut really short and see what happens. The wig hasn't come yet but I might just wear a headscarf anyway.

I felt quite well after the chemo, so I popped into the hospice and had lunch with the day patients. That was a mistake. I brought it all back up again this evening. I wasn't sick once during the first treatment cycle, just nauseated. Next time I won't have lunch! I slept this afternoon and am spending this evening in bed. It's Tuesday so I wanted Nick to go to chess but he has very wisely left some sweets on the doorstep with a note asking any trick-or-treaters not to knock. We wouldn't normally do this; this year's an exception!

November 2006

Tuesday 7 November
Discovering what it is like to be a patient

I'm never going to be a completely normal patient, I know too much about the medication and am also surrounded by those who can give me advice; however, that doesn't mean I am not experiencing some of the horrors of treatment. My second dose of chemotherapy was on 31 October.

On Sunday morning (5 November) I went to the hospice. I was greeted by Jane, the community cancer nurse specialist; she informed me that I was looking tired and I looked as if I had just stopped dexamethasone. This, of course was very accurate and I was tired, lacking energy; my mood was low. I was still suffering some nausea and was also very constipated.

Sleep had been very difficult because of the effects of high dose dexamethasone. I had eventually taken half a 3.75 mg zopiclone sleeping tablet at 2 a.m. but this hadn't helped.

I have never been as constipated in my life as I was by Sunday afternoon. By early evening I was becoming so agitated that I couldn't sit, I couldn't relax and I certainly couldn't concentrate on reading. Two suppositories and an attempt at a rather crude manual evacuation later (fortunately, I had gloves, glycerine suppositories and lubricant available), and I was a bit more comfortable but knew it was only the start!

I realised the importance of being able to take myself to bed in the early evening rather than trying to sit downstairs. Bed rest can be very therapeutic, but patients need to be able to choose to be up or in bed. This is a real problem for more disabled patients, relying on carers to get them to bed. Just being able to rest properly with my feet up in bed is so much more comfortable. It must be so frustrating for patients when they become too weak to move around and pull themselves back up the bed. At least I could keep changing positions until I was comfortable, and I had to get comfortable to help resolve some of the agitation. Fortunately, the previous day I had managed to find a large, firm cushion to act as a backrest to prop myself up in bed, so I could try to read in bed.

Falling asleep for a short nap turned out to be what I actually needed. It appears to be important to allow my body to dictate its needs rather than forcing myself to keep to a normal routine. I certainly would not have coped going to church in the evening, nor would anyone else have coped with me. I even slept in spite of the fireworks!

At 10 p.m. I was awake and feeling better – anxious, though, that I would manage to sleep during the night, preferably without a sleeping tablet; anxious, also, that I had to be up for surgery in the morning, but still with the only partially resolved problem of constipation.

Sunday 12 November

I woke at 6 a.m. this morning feeling quite refreshed. It's now day 13 of my second cycle of chemotherapy so I'm beginning to feel more normal again. From a medical point of view, observing side-effects of the drugs, most of the problems appear to be the same this cycle as last. It's worth documenting them so I am even better prepared next cycle. I've been told I will struggle more later on. People keep sounding very reassuring. 'When you have the next lot you will be half-way through.' Well, yes, OK but the tedium of going through another three cycles and another three doses of side-effects will still have to be endured.

Physical side-effects

Nausea: I have only vomited once – in the evening following my second dose of chemotherapy. This was my own fault. I ate a lovely lunch after having chemo in the morning. I had been feeling well enough to eat but then suffered 'delayed gastric emptying'. Although I had had intravenous granesetron and oral metoclopramide, the nausea increased, but after I vomited I felt so much better and slept.

We really must remember at the hospice not necessarily to rush in with anti-emetics after someone has been sick, with a high obstruction or delayed gastric emptying, as vomiting may be the only cure, and then the symptoms resolve.

The day after chemo I needed granesetron 1mg plus three doses of metoclopramide 10mg to control nausea, but managed to eat small meals. I developed waves of nausea by 10 p.m. which settled with the third dose of metoclopramide and bed rest.

Day 3 – Thursday – of the first cycle I felt (and apparently looked) rough on arrival at work in the hospice. My colleagues suggested I took a further dose of granesetron rather than relying solely on metoclopramide.

During the first cycle, I coped without granesetron on day 4 but had a dose on the Friday of the second cycle. I had to drive to the surgery and see patients all morning, I didn't want to risk being ill. The inevitable consequence of this was severe constipation – worse than the first cycle.

Really potent, new drugs are of great benefit but may well have very unpleasant side-effects. Patients need to be warned and the side-effects adequately anticipated. I may try to cope on day four without granesetron, next cycle and see how I manage.

During both cycles I managed to stop anti-emetics completely by day six to seven. The dexamethasone, prescribed to avoid late-onset nausea, mid-cycle, clearly works but again, not without side-effects (see mood).

Constipation

I now know how awful severe constipation can be. It is so uncomfortable. It made me agitated, restless, and unable to concentrate or relax.

If agitation is due to constipation in the terminal stage of life, addressing this should be considered rather than just treating with sedation. We successfully relieve agitation by catheterising a patient as necessary, but do we remember constipation?

Next cycle I need to take a stronger laxative before I become constipated but also consider reducing the amount of granesetron

I take, as the symptoms were more manageable during the first cycle.

Monday 13 November
Laughter

Yesterday was full of laughter. Yesterday I even woke up laughing! I lay in bed thinking about one of our regular day hospice patients who had been an in-patient for a couple of weeks. He had suddenly started feeling better and on Thursday (9 November) I was told he had spent the previous evening at home and thoroughly enjoyed himself. He was keen to prove he was ready to go home. He already knew I was ill and even if he didn't, it's pretty obvious to hospice patients that a doctor, wearing a hat to disguise the fact she's losing her hair, is having chemotherapy. He had also noticed that I like to sit down on a chair when I am talking to patients on the ward round, to improve communication. Really listening and watching the patient to assess their needs being the most important aspect of providing quality palliative care.

This patient, however, demonstrated another important use of this communication tool. As I approached his bed he was sitting in the only chair next to his bed. He immediately stood up and said 'I will get you your chair, doctor.' If the palliative care patient is well enough to fetch the doctor her chair he is probably well enough to go home. It was this little incident that had made me laugh on waking up.

At church several people said how well I looked. Most of the time I feel quite well and relaxed as well. Should I be worried when people imply that I am looking better than I have for a long time?

In the afternoon we saw Marian Elizabeth performing in the new play by Alex Viac at the Old Red Lion Theatre in Angel. I thought she acted beautifully and the short play *Waste Disposal* was frequently very funny. The theatre was full and, being the upper room of a pub, a very intimate space. After the performance, Alex the writer came and sat next to me and thanked me for laughing. He said that he was sure I had been the first to laugh and one person laughing gives permission for others to laugh, too. There had been very little laughter during the first two performances but he was genuinely delighted that he had written a comedy, although he said he hadn't realised he had!

Laughter transforms things.

For me, laughter, especially in consultations, is a vital part of the treatment process. A patient reflected today that her mood was lifting now that she was on antidepressants and her sense of humour has returned. Another patient, today, brought me in a funny poem to read that a friend had written her fifteen years ago following her mastectomy, to cheer her up. She checked first that I was in the mood for a laugh and then gave me the poem. She said that at the time of her diagnosis she found a light-hearted approach was what she needed. Some of her friends were quite shocked feeling that solemnity was more appropriate. I told her that Joe, in the consulting room next door, had been very relieved to hear my laughter through the wall, as a sign that I was coping!

More than a decade ago, I was told at my previous practice, by the woman who was then my practice manager, that I didn't take work seriously enough. It was clear, in the context of our discussion, that she didn't like me smiling or my laughter. She was profoundly wrong and was probably very jealous of my relaxed, open, confident and friendly approach. What she said that day was extremely hurtful and had a significant effect on my confidence. If she had aimed to demoralise me, she succeeded. Fortunately, my sense of humour is welcomed and warmly acknowledged as necessary at the hospice and at my present practice.

Why is it you have to be ill to receive gorgeous letters? Often people don't write letters until someone has died; at least I'm here to read them! I received a gorgeous letter the other day that brought tears to my eyes.

Tuesday 14 November

I am due to have another scan this evening to assess the progress of my chemotherapy. I really can't tell if things are getting better. There is still a lump there but it feels less obvious. The trouble is I am struggling to remember what it felt like initially. Once I had had the biopsy it became huge due to a large haematoma (bruise) and its basic shape was completely masked. It has become smaller since then, but I wonder if that is just the ant-inflammatory effect of two courses of dexamethasone, rather than the chemotherapy itself. Ultrasound will be much more conclusive.

Thursday 16 November
Coping with bad news

Everyone has been saying I am doing well, coping so well with the diagnosis and treatment. Friends at work have used words like 'amazing' to describe how I've been a great example to others. Whether it has been right to try to work or not, only time will tell but I know I have gained from it.

Unfortunately, the scan on Tuesday evening picked up a second tumour in my breast. I knew my type of breast cancer was more difficult to identify using ultrasound scans but I hadn't expected this. The chemotherapy doesn't seem to have done much and now we know I have two tumours anyway, I have no choice, I need a mastectomy, and within days.

Coming to terms with the nature of the operation is a real struggle, trying to imagine how I will look, trying to decide what to say to people. Should I say that I will be having a mastectomy? Do I want people thinking of me with only one breast? What an awful thought! Talking about it is in fact the way I cope, and the way I find easiest to manage the situation.

Tuesday 21 November

Things have moved very fast: I'm having a mastectomy tomorrow.

There was a fantastically reassuring message on our answer machine after a meal out on Friday, from Richard, my anaesthetist – I wonder how often that happens!

I had a great day on Saturday going to the history of medicine course, seeing Marian and going to the matinee of *Porgy and Bess* at the Savoy. It was fantastic. I realised how well I was feeling as I managed to run up the Strand to the Savoy to get the tickets. Ten days ago in London I had struggled to climb the steps to cross the river to Waterloo and had to walk very slowly across the bridge.

By Sunday morning at church I realised that I needed to be honest with myself and others, and admitted that I was scared. It was good to have prayer and receive communion.

Even when scared it's great to have a sense of humour. During the final prayer – 'We offer you are souls and bodies to be a living sacrifice...' – a picture of me on the operating table flashed through my mind. At least we pray *'living* sacrifice'.

I took my last surgery yesterday for a long time.

Before beginning surgery Sally, who works there, told me about a dream she had had during the night about me starting as a larva and her being escorted around an insect house and eventually me emerging as a butterfly. She felt sure it was a promise that I would be OK.

My penultimate patient, John is waiting for an operation too. He asked me how I felt (about having surgery) so I said I was scared to which he replied, 'It's reassuring to know you're scared; so am I.' I explained that I hadn't had a major operation before and he said he hadn't either.

I had my pre-op assessment in the afternoon. Time really dragged but at least my white cell count was adequate. I realised that I would have really struggled to cope if I had had to wait another week. At least going into a private hospital guarantees I will have a bed tomorrow and I will have the operation. No further delays.

I lay in bed this morning praying for our daughters, and praising the Lord for their gifts. Again, I felt so grateful and thankful that they are using their gifts of music and drama to glorify the Lord. I'm particularly proud (am I allowed to feel pride?) that Rachel is being encouraged again to play her cello for worship within her new church family.

We had a long day shopping at Milton Keynes today. Excellent distraction therapy! We were meant to be doing Christmas shopping but instead I bought a lovely cosy, cream coloured dressing gown, some slippers and bed socks. Most important of all, I was measured for bras. The fitter was a young girl, but she was very sensible. She advised me to get a soft sports bra that wouldn't rub the scar. I told her I was having surgery but she wasn't a specially trained fitter for ladies post-mastectomy, just a wise young woman. Believe it or not, that was the first time I had ever had a proper fitting. I was wearing completely the wrong size cup! The breast care nurse asked me to get measured so they could get the correct prosthesis for me.

Wednesday 22 November

Today's the day. At least I know that when I get to the Chiltern Hospital at lunchtime there will be a bed for me and I will have my operation. I'm scared, I want to run away, but I am so fortunate to have private insurance for this part of my treatment. I may be scared but my mind and my body are prepared. I do not know how my patients cope when they get to the hospital and the operation is cancelled, or they ring up from home in the morning to discover there is no bed for them. To me that would be torture. This is my first major operation. I don't want it, but there is one thing for certain: I have got to go through with it, and at the end of the day I will have lost a breast. If I had to cope with the possibility that I might have to go through the preparation process all over again, the uncertainty would be unbearable.

My first port of call today was the radioisotope department at Wycombe General Hospital so that I can have a sentinel node biopsy during surgery. The first lymph node in the chain of axillary nodes draining the right breast is to be removed. If there is tumour in this node, further surgery is required to remove the other nodes, if not, we can assume the rest are clear.

Thursday 23 November

It's all over! It wasn't easy doing a wee in the middle of the night with a drip in my left hand, a drain in my right side and inflatable socks rhythmically compressing and releasing my calf muscles to prevent a deep vein thrombosis. The nurses were great. I told them there was no way I would be able to wee in a bedpan. (I knew that from past experience of childbirth!) They helped me out onto a commode; a mammoth task for which I was extremely grateful.

This morning the drip came down and I ate an excellent breakfast. I am amazed I have had no nausea and I have had one anti-inflammatory for pain. That's all. I haven't needed to have any morphine to relieve my pain, which is fantastic as it would have caused constipation. Richard, my anaesthetist, gave me an intrapleural nerve block which is such good pain relief during surgery that, apparently, I did not need heavy sedation during the operation, but, of course I wasn't aware of it at all. The nerve block still seems to be providing me with good analgesia. It is great to be able to move around the bed. I really struggled to move with the drip one side and the drain the other.

There are advantages and disadvantages to being a private patient in my own single room. In the middle of the night I did feel rather isolated even though I knew I could call for a nurse, but Marian is coming to look after me today so that is very special.

Yesterday, when we arrived at the Chiltern, I had to wait longer than I had expected before surgery because I was second on the list for the afternoon. When Alan came to see me before the operation we discussed the consent. I initially signed to consent to right mastectomy and sentinel node biopsy. Just before Alan left the room it crossed my mind to ask him if it would be worth agreeing to anything else. We both decided it would be wise for him to remove more nodes if he felt they might be cancerous and that might spare me any further surgery. I was being realistic. Let's face it, it is eight weeks since I first noticed the lump and the chemo I have had has, at best, been of minimal benefit, so spread to the lymph nodes is quite likely. In the event Alan removed eight nodes.

Once they were ready for me in theatre I don't remember much except that I was surprised and amused that I walked there. Well, there was no reason why not – I wasn't drowsy. Pre-meds seem to be a thing of the past, but I hadn't expected it. In my day, patients would go on a trolley or at least in a wheelchair. I put my slippers and dressing gown on and had to follow the attendant. In my head I was humming *The March to the Scaffold* from Berlioz's *Symphonie Fantastique*. It seemed most appropriate. I can recall a large clock on the wall that I could read even without my glasses. It was approximately 4 p.m. Richard numbed the back of my hand prior to inserting a cannula. I told him I thought that was extremely kind but rather unnecessary. I don't numb the area first when I'm putting drips up! The next thing I remember is reassuring voices calling to me as I came round. I tried to speak. I was incoherent. My voice was slow, deep and husky and very strange. I noticed it was about 7.30 p.m.

Nick was waiting for me in the room with what appeared to be a bunch of cabbages on stalks. Actually it is a very attractive and rather unusual flower arrangement, better appreciated in the light of day! My voice came back very quickly over night, too. Richard told me that I was a good patient and easy to anaesthetise. That is really reassuring and very nice to know. I knew I was in good hands but it is nice to know I didn't cause him extra stress. However just because I was easy to anaesthetise doesn't mean I want to go through the process again!

Friday 24 November

I had a lovely long chat with the breast care nurse today. She has fitted me with a soft prosthesis so that when I leave the hospital (hopefully tomorrow) I will look symmetrical.

The physiotherapists have also shown me some exercises. I had lots of visits yesterday including two clergy, which was lovely, but today has been much quieter. However, the food is great and my bowels are working. I'm still pain-free! Great news, though: Rachel is coming home for the weekend to look after me, and Marian will be home on Sunday.

Saturday 25 November.

It poured with rain this morning but Alan came to see me once it had stopped and I was told the drain could come out and I could go home after lunch.

Sunday 26 November.

I went to our local community church this morning with Marian and Rachel. It was great to be there and people were amazed. I went to church with Nick in the evening. It was good to thank people for praying and to praise God, even if I have to sit for most of the service.

Monday 27 November
Post-op recovery

I walked back from Jansel Square, the local shops, today which didn't seem to over-tax me at all. I don't think I could have walked there and back. I might try going to the hospice tomorrow, though, to see people – not sure.

I'm trying to get used to wearing a breast prosthesis. This was something I hadn't thought about at all until just before the operation. In fact, I really hadn't given it much thought when seeing patients with breast cancer either. I'm still acutely aware that I keep checking I look symmetrical. I'm glad I can joke about it, otherwise I might cry. Chris, my friend with a below-knee amputation, was a wonderful role model as someone with a sense of humour about having a prosthesis. I also keep chuckling to myself about the alcoholic who I've seen a couple of times in the police cells who when arrested 'drunk and disorderly' and helped down to the cells clutching his artificial leg in one hand declares to everyone that he is 'legless'.

Losing a leg is so much bigger than losing a breast but probably less embarrassing.

I want to try to show people I still have my sense of humour and I am still feeling positive about all this. How can I do this in an email or a text message? Is it OK to make jokes about being lopsided? Is that too embarrassing?

I hope people don't think I am trying to prove I'm super-woman, because I am definitely not; in fact I'm trying to learn to slow down but I have to be me, I have to do what feels right.

I really wanted to go to church yesterday to worship and let people see that their prayers had been answered. Mary especially had been praying for a good anaesthetic and good pain control so she saw her prayer had been answered in a wonderful way.

December 2006

Sunday 3 December

I'm feeling rather uncomfortable and irritable this evening. It is rather sore under my right arm.

Spiritual reflection

I had a wonderful walk yesterday along the canal at Marsworth. I had really wanted to go for a walk as I had missed my times of reflection and prayer whilst enjoying God's creation. I had managed to time my afternoon nap to give me time to go for a walk before it became too dark. I wish it didn't get dark so early! The afternoon was beautiful but the sun was already low in the sky as I walked around Startops reservoir. There were so many great-crested grebes on the reservoir. As I walked alone alongside the canal, I began to feel refreshed as I reflected, watched and prayed. I pondered some words that David the chaplain had said when I had popped into the hospice on Thursday. At the time I had said I wasn't feeling very positive. (I had only just received the histology following my mastectomy, and was trying to come to terms with it.) Very gently, David had reminded me that Jesus – the very human Jesus – had struggled emotionally, not only in the Garden of Gethsemane, but at other times as well. Struggling is OK; not feeling positive is OK; I need to be real and honest with my feelings. After all, am I holier than Jesus? Certainly not! This was much more helpful for me, at that moment, than the comment others have made that I had got to maintain a positive mental attitude to maximise healing potential. Fortunately the great Healer in whom I put my faith understands my mood.

As I walked I reflected on how I tended to focus on Jesus the Son of God in the 'I Am' passages in John's gospel, and Jesus the High Priest in Hebrews, but hadn't focused on Jesus the person; the very human being. Throughout this illness I have been saying, 'I need to be myself' and do what I feel I need, but I was still expecting to cope well all the time. I can honestly say I had been coping and I had surprised myself how much easier it had been than I expected. I had attributed this to people's prayer, but was feeling guilty that my mood had dropped, in spite of this. David and I had talked about answers to prayer. I know the Lord is with me all the time but some of the time I am more aware of this than others. I was reminded of this today. It was nearly dark, as again I walked along the canal at Broughton with the full moon reflected on the relatively still waters of the canal. The moon was much higher in the sky than it had been eight weeks ago when I had just been diagnosed, but it was still shining in the canal. The clouds covered the moon for a short time. I knew it was still there but it was hidden. God is always there but may seem hidden.

Yesterday as I walked by the canal reflecting on my vulnerability as a human being and praying I remembered the words of psalm 23: 'He leads me beside still waters, He restores my soul'. I had missed my walks and began to realise that that was exactly what was happening. Through having time on my own to be quiet, to enjoy God's creation and praise Him for its beauty, the Lord was 'restoring my soul'.

Monday 4 December
Reflection on histology and prognosis

Was it wise to obtain my full histology off the hospital computer?

Alan had told me of the eight nodes removed three lymph nodes contained malignant cells, but now I could see it in black and white.

Was it wise to do a Google search last night to establish a prognosis from the information? Was it going to plunge me into depression?

I slept quite well last night once I was comfortable. I hadn't expected to sleep but whilst lying in bed I had started to think about other medical statistics; risk factors for disease. I regularly tell patients about their cardiovascular risk. I often have to tell men that their risk of a heart attack or stroke in the next ten years is 30 per cent or more. At this point, of course we can prescribe medication and encourage lifestyle changes to improve things,, but if they go away and think about the information, it must bring them face to face with their own mortality. I'm not much worse off.

Obtaining one interpretation of my histology is helpful – 50–64 per cent of women in my situation live at least ten years after diagnosis. It's not brilliant but it could be worse. It will help me discuss my future with colleagues. It will help me to be realistic.

The other bit of helpful information is that most recurrences occur in the first two years, but of course breast cancer can recur after fifteen or more years. That doesn't matter so much. It is what to do for the next few (working) years that matter, at present.

I have three jobs with contracts and a fourth source of income – Mental Health Act assessments – if I want it. Is this what I want to spend the next few years doing? Is this the best use of my time? Are there other things that are more important, more enjoyable, and more worthwhile? What am I really finding satisfying at present? In which of the jobs can I give most? Where am I most effective or useful?

Over the last six years I have given my time to support my colleagues and to help maintain rotas with out-of-hours work, etc. Supporting others is probably what I have found most rewarding but partly because I feel needed.

It is time to say that I can't go on doing all these things but I feel I need to present a case. Having these statistics will help me, even though it may sound rather morbid – as if I am giving up.

Tuesday 5 December

I went into day hospice today, not as a doctor but as a patient. I have started making a mosaic. I have always wanted to 'have a go' and now I'm ill I can achieve that ambition. It's of a crane (the bird!). It's going to take many weeks.

Friday 8 December

Today, I have spent some time typing up my handwritten reflections produced whilst on holiday in Plymouth, earlier in my illness. It was good to think again about my walk along the canal and the full moon. Last weekend, I sat on the Broughton lock gate after the sun had set on Sunday afternoon. The moon was high in the sky with its light reflecting on the water but the water was not so still, as it had been raining so hard, the water was rushing over the top of the gates. It was eight weeks since that special evening, but of course the sun now sets so early in the day. Trying to fit in a walk during daylight after an afternoon sleep is quite hard. As I looked at the moon it was clear that the impact of the moon rising two months ago could not have been repeated this month, as the moon rose during daylight.

Today I have really appreciated the kindness of some of our church home group members. Tonight's supper was provided, quite unexpectedly, by Alison who brought a chilli con carne over, yesterday. I have found it quite difficult to ask for things. It is so much easier when they just arrive. It was so good to have something that could be heated up the following day, giving me time to plan.

I am struggling to do more than one thing a day. I went to a meeting today at Wendover police station but yesterday I had three visitors. Lorna and her husband came in the morning and Alison in the afternoon, after my sleep. I coped, and enjoyed the time, but really it was a bit too much.

It was lovely talking to them all. Lorna shared her experience of chemotherapy and how to cope with constipation. Alison shared her experience of being bullied at work. This is such a difficult problem. It was good to be able to share with her.

I showed her Philippians. 1: 29: 'For it has been granted to you that for the sake of Christ you should not only believe in him but also suffer for his sake.' This was a verse that had taken me a while to find. I remembered a preacher talking about the Greek root of the verb translated 'granted' being charis. This means 'grace' as a noun but 'to give a gift' as the verb. I couldn't remember which letter of St Paul it came from, but eventually found it with the help of a concordance. (Alison has been studying ancient Greek recently and I studied it at school.) I then looked up the Greek in my Greek New Testament and was puzzled as the word didn't look right. At this point, much to my amazement, I realised I had picked up a misprint in the Greek! The word was echaristhe *which had been translated 'it was granted' but in fact should read 'given as a gift'. And what was this gift? The gift is 'to suffer'. This has been an enormous comfort to me, and it was great to share it with a friend who has just been studying ancient Greek, and had also experienced suffering.*

Another friend from the church, Margaret, had visited on Wednesday and I shared that with her too. She is retired now and always seems very busy, but is looking at how she should best use her time. She said she found chatting with me was a real help, and Alison found encouragement, so perhaps this is something good that is coming out of my illness. I have more time for my friends.

Saturday 9 December

I am beginning to feel more normal again but I still need a sleep after lunch. It is still taking me until 10.a.m. to get up and dressed. I have managed to go shopping and go to a concert today. It was an amazing concert with the Balanescu quartet and friends, (of *University Challenge* music fame). I feel really privileged to have heard them perform, especially in Aylesbury. I'm certainly not ready to travel up to London for the day. I am still very uncomfortable under my right arm, by evening.

My concentration is improving and I am managing to spend more time working on the computer and reading. I am encouraged, and then remember that in eleven days' time I start chemotherapy all over again. As doctors, we do demand an awful lot from patients. You start to feel better, so you are hit again by the next round of therapy. I am only just beginning to appreciate what an ordeal we inflict on patients. This is fine when the hope is possible 'cure', but what about those who have no possibility of anything more than temporary palliation? How much suffering can a patient endure for a short reprieve? Lorna was right to ask the question: 'Is it worth it?' It was good to see that she is feeling well, and looking forward to Christmas. After all, she hadn't expected to be alive at Christmas.

People are so kind. Shirley has taken my ironing home with her and will return it tomorrow. I could really have done it myself, but it would have meant leaving other things undone. I am just starting to learn to receive from others rather, than trying to give all the time. It's a very hard lesson to learn, and I still feel guilty that I am not spending enough time reflecting and typing this journal.

I want to start writing up my own past experience of suffering at the hand of bullies, in the dysfunctional practice, but I don't know where to start. I don't need to start at the beginning, but it is having the courage to start at all. I've got the time at the moment, so I really need to make an effort.

Monday 18 December
Manchester

We went to a carol service yesterday evening where Rachel was playing in the orchestra. We had left her to rehearse after lunch. She then played for an afternoon and the evening service. They only rehearsed the once and she was asked to play a solo. It was very special. We also had a good chat with one of her pastors. She was so supportive. It was good to tell her about my cancer.

We spent the morning looking round the Lowry exhibition in Salford. It was wonderful.

We picked Rachel up form her school and drove over to my aunt's. Rachel's completed her first teaching practice in Manchester. I'm very pleased with her.

It was really good to see my Aunt Gladwys and cousins, and to meet little Phoebe for the first time. She is quite an extrovert. It was a sad time though, as James died last week. We chatted about James's funeral. I'm so sad we won't be there as I have to be back in Aylesbury for my first dose of the new chemotherapy. They wanted the funeral to be tomorrow but it can't take place until Wednesday.

James celebrated his eighteenth birthday, even though both he and his brother Daniel have Duchenne muscular dystrophy. I am so impressed with my aunt; she gave her grandsons such a special life.

Tuesday 19 December

I had to take 16 mg of dexamethasone today before having docetaxol tomorrow. It's to try to prevent me from having an allergic reaction to the chemo, because it's made from yew tree pine needles. I really didn't want to. I had enough side-effects from 8 mg dexamethasone a day. This is twice as much. What on earth will it do to my mood and my weight?

Reflection on the journey to come

We returned from Manchester today with Rachel plus her new guitar. It was a good long weekend, especially meeting Debra Green at Ivy Cottage and my cousin Jacx and her very lively four-year-old daughter Phoebe. It is so obvious that Phoebe is Rachel and Marian's cousin!

Going away helped me forget what is about to happen, but taking the 16 mg of Dexamethasone today ensured the reality of chemotherapy sank home. I became very anxious on the way home, and just wanted to curl up in bed this afternoon. All I wanted to do was run away. I am so glad Rachel will be there with me tomorrow for my first dose of docetaxol. Phyllis, GP Allan's widow, may be there as well, working as a volunteer. I received some beautiful flowers from her today. It is wonderful to see how she is now flourishing again, after Allan died. His death was so hard for her.

I know I should not be anxious about anything, but trust God and the doctors involved, but I can understand why people are frightened. It is a huge ordeal that I am going through. I am glad I start tomorrow – before Christmas – as it would have ruined Boxing Day thinking about chemo on the next day, and there is no point putting it off longer than I have to.

This afternoon I started to think again about the lady who decided not to have conventional treatment six years ago. If only I could have said to her: 'I'm scared too, but I am going to follow the experts' advice.' It really makes me angry – especially at the moment – to think how she was deceived by those who gave her 'false hope' by offering alternative therapies which were easier, required less adjustments to her routine and, at the time, less pain. Complementary therapies can be really beneficial alongside conventional treatment but alternative therapies shouldn't replace conventional treatment.

I'm sure it was fear that stopped her having surgery and chemo: fear of the unknown, fear of the cancer (try and ignore it) and fear of pain, so she opted for the easier route. This route was said to offer a 'cure' but without any scientific evidence behind it. It cost so much money but where was the accountability of the healer? Where was the alternative therapist when she died?

Maybe there is a parallel here. When Jesus said 'Deny yourselves, take up your cross and follow me,' he wasn't offering an easy life – a prosperity gospel – but he does offer the gift of eternal life; the right to become children of God. Following Jesus may not be easy but it leads to the truth. Jesus fully accounts for everything he says. The alternative path may seem better and simpler but can deceive.

Wednesday 20 December

Rachel accompanied me to the chemotherapy unit. I have to take a further 16 mg dexamethasone today and the same tomorrow, and then I stop them.

I am so glad Rachel came with me. The process was quite uneventful; the infusion went very smoothly. My nurse is a friend of Rachel's, so they had a good chat.

Friday 22 December

I haven't had any dexamethasone today and my mood has dropped.

This evening I don't feel like doing much at all, but it is important I make a note of my feelings, so I know what to expect next time. Nausea has not been a great problem, so I have had metoclopramide, but not granesetron today.

We went to the practice lunchtime 'Christmas do' and I coped! I had a good chat with our midwife, Paula. She's doing a degree and has been keeping a journal that she is finding very helpful. We talked about the need to be more 'mature' to produce adequate reflection!

I lay in bed last night trying to get to sleep, and thought about the statistics. Using a computer program, we calculated I have a 61.8 per cent chance of being alive in ten years or getting to sixty, or reaching retirement age. I then started mulling over the fact that my tumour was a lobular carcinoma. Only 10–15 per cent of breast cancers are lobular tumours, and a small number of these are multi-focal. Also, only 20–30 per cent of breast tumours don't respond to the first-line chemotherapy – FEC – but mine didn't. Oh well – these are only statistics.

Christmas Day

Mum is due to go in for her knee replacement at the end of the week. I haven't seen her since I was diagnosed. She hasn't been able to drive over to see me, and I have been too weak to travel to see her.

We cooked the turkey last night, packed it in the car and drove over to Beckenham to spend Christmas Day with her. For the first time in years I missed the midnight communion. I needed to sleep. Marian came with us to Mum's but Rachel was already there. I had a rest in the afternoon and Nick gave me two very practical presents: an electric steamer and a gadget for removing bottle and jar lids. He has obviously been thinking about how weak I am likely to get!

Boxing Day

This entry should be entitled 'learning how to live when your husband has a cold and you have just had chemo'!

I had far too much to eat yesterday. It took me ages to get off to sleep. Nick had to sleep in the spare bedroom as we were keeping each other awake. I was getting a lot of neck ache and pain in my throat and ears. Is this the start of a viral infection? Am I going to cope with this if I don't have many white cells? Am I getting a temperature?

I was tossing and turning I just could not get comfortable. I couldn't find a position to lie in that was comfortable enough for me to relax.

Before people die they often become agitated. I'm not surprised, if I can't get comfortable in bed at this stage, even when I can roll over without difficulty, it must be awful for a dying patient who is so weak he can't move around in the bed, without help.

Wednesday 27 December

I got some lovely presents from patients. They are from people who have had difficulties in the past. They all have their own stories. It has been a real privilege to hear their stories; some have shared their deepest frustrations with me. They found my illness hard but have found a way of showing their gratitude.

It would be so much easier to write up my diary resting in bed rather than sitting at a desk. I think it is time to look in the sales for a laptop!

Thursday 28 December

I started crying before I went to sleep last night. I was reflecting on a few thoughts for another informal talk at church. I realised that it is impossible to separate completely my thoughts about my experience at my previous practice, and what is happening at the moment. Although the events are years apart they are both very much part of 'my story', and involve suffering. However, I began to realise last night, that what is happening now may be helping to heal some of the wounds inflicted on me then, which I have either suppressed, tried to ignore, or even strived to adjust to inappropriately. I decided to try to put thoughts neatly into another short 'testimony' for Sunday. I suppose it is rather like the 'play within the play' that Shakespeare was so fond of; it is impossible to separate the two, without losing some of the meaning and purpose of the story. (For more reflections on my time at that practice, see the chapter entitled 'Play within the play'.)

Reflection for Sunday evening service

One of the huge 'advantages' of becoming very seriously ill and taking sick leave, rather than, for example, having an accident and not living to tell the tale, is that you get to read the lovely things people write about you in letters and cards. In fact, what I am about to say could really be entitled 'A tale of two letters', or 'it was the best of times, it was the worst of times'.

Earlier this year, as a result of the philosophy and ethics diploma I was taking, I again became quite preoccupied by the events that took place when the girls were little, and I realised that there were still a lot of wounds that I had suppressed that really needed healing.

When I started working as a police surgeon (long before the police started to call us FMEs or forensic medical examiners), I got to know both the wives of my male colleagues, who in their turn have both sent me incredibly significant letters.

I received the one from Mrs C, who worked as the practice manager, a year after I ceased working with them. I carried a copy around with me for a long, long time until I had my handbag stolen. I had not carried another significant letter around with me since, until I received a letter from Phyllis, Allan's widow, recently. It was a great privilege to look after Allan as a patient before he died, to gently persuade him to stop being a doctor and allow me and my team to take over (something I'm struggling to do myself just at the moment!) It has also been wonderful to support Phyllis and see her flourishing again.

As I said, this is the tale of two letters. The first letter served as a reminder to me of what I had been through: the dreadful loneliness of being branded the enemy, of being spat at, demonised and shouted at, and – worst of all – just not good enough for them because they said that I didn't take the work seriously enough.

Even though it's years later, I realise that that is still getting to me. You see, I do laugh and joke during consultations, and with the rest of the team at work; it's part of my style of consultation, and that was being undermined as being unprofessional and inappropriate. The very nature of my practice was being questioned by the practice manager. The letter itself said it all; at least it proved that I hadn't imagined what I went through. Among other things, it stated that I was the 'nastiest, most vindictive and wicked person to have ever walked this earth'. I didn't take that too much to heart; it was the insidious drip, drip, drip of the lesser accusations that took their toll. Incidentally, I heard from a patient, after I left, that she had been informed that they had asked me to leave because I was too religious. I had certainly questioned their ethical standards.

So, what about the other letter, the one I now carry around with me? The one I would not have received if I hadn't been ill; those beautiful healing words!

'Hazel, your lovely smile will take you through the next few months. You may be unaware how we patients feel when your face lights up with your smile. It is how I always think of you and others have said the same.'

What a contrast; two letters, two doctors' wives, one trying to encourage and build up, the other trying to destroy.

Friday 29 December

Mum had her knee replacement today. I'm really pleased that she was able to speak to me and was enjoying her evening meal. Certainly, recovery after anaesthetic seems to be much quicker these days!

I have caught Nick's cold and cough, and my temperature has been up to 37.6°C. I don't know if I overreacted, but I decided to get my blood count checked to see whether I am neutropenic, so at risk of severe sepsis. I'm mid-cycle – nine days since I had chemo and unfortunately I have 0.1 neutrophils. Docetaxol certainly does destroy my neutrophils! I need to keep a close eye on my temperature, and complete my course of the antibiotic ciprofloxacin. Maybe I overreacted, but with the three-day weekend and bank holiday coming up, I wanted to share the responsibility for my management; to be a patient rather than a doctor. At least I, as a doctor, now know the extent of the neutropenia I will develop with each cycle of this chemotherapy. It may assist me in my decision making about working within general practice during the next few months.

The other day, I had a look at the docetaxol patient information leaflet to clarify the side-effects and interactions. One clinician in the US on another website stated that patients shouldn't drink alcohol when on docetaxol. I wondered if the leaflet would clarify this. It didn't, but as it can cause hepatitis (inflammation of the liver), particularly in the first cycle, this may be the reason. As I had been drinking alcohol, but have also noticed a very significant tachycardia (fast heart rate), making it very difficult to sleep, I have decided to abstain for the rest of this cycle, anyway.

I have established that docetaxol is made from the 'renewable biomass of yew tree pine needles'. The drug firm seemed to need to emphasise that they weren't damaging trees, but since the downloadable 'leaflet' runs to fifty-five pages, this seems rather ironic! It seems rather comforting that a product from the yew tree, that great guardian of many of our church graveyards, is playing such an important part in determining my life expectancy.

January 2007

Monday 1 January

I have been reflecting further on last night's evening service.

There was no planned evening service for New Year's Eve but a decision was made during the morning to have an informal service. I had had a rough night – waking up coughing on three occasions and needing to sit upright to stop coughing. I read most of a book loaned me by Margaret during the night. During that time, I suddenly thought that there would be a service after all, and as I had partly prepared a talk, it might be right to say something. I shared this with Roger at church in the morning, and he said nothing else had been prepared!

Eighteen people came to the service, which, for me, was just right. To present my talk as the focus of a service was certainly not what I had expected. (We are usually just invited to say something, informally, at the start of the service. The sermon is separate.) However, it was clear that people were really listening. I found myself emphasising the phrase 'the loneliness of being branded the enemy' all those years ago, and the beginning of psychological healing through reading Phyllis's letter.

We then sang the chosen worship songs. One I had never sung before but the words were beautiful – all about being chosen and loved by the Father. It beautifully summed up what I had said.

This morning at the beginning of the new year I read a beautiful chapter by Nouwen on blessing, on being blessed and giving blessings. He talked about the importance of affirming people, just as Phyllis had done in her letter, clearly expressing what I mean to her and others, and what is special. Marian is very good at this in cards, etc, and I spoke to Rachel, who said she had spent the morning sending people text messages to bless them at the beginning of the new year. My daughters obviously have a better idea of the importance of affirmation than I had at that age!

Affirming qualities in people is important, as those things that mean most to other people, the person herself may not be aware of. As Phyllis said: 'You may be unaware....'

Tuesday 2 January

I slept well last night, only woke up once coughing but settled quickly. Much better than the last two nights, and probably rather better than Nick who hasn't had a course of antibiotics!

This was the first morning since my operation that I felt like getting up and on with housework at a reasonable hour – 7.30 a.m.!

I got on and did the ironing, and wrote up some reflections, prior to going to day hospice for 10.30 a.m.

Pat was on her own in day hospice as the patients don't return until tomorrow, after the Christmas break. She allowed me to do my mosaic anyway. It was really rewarding and therapeutic working on the mosaic for three hours, talking to Pat and Helen and Debbie. I was really pleased with my level of concentration. I am definitely feeling better.

My improvement prompted me to contact Nick the senior FME to arrange to do a few daytime sessions of police work, covering Aylesbury. Rosemary, our police work administrator, was thrilled to find me well enough even to consider doing some work; she is so caring!

Mum is doing well post-op following her knee replacement, except she is very constipated (I know what that is like!). Marian visited her today. I am so pleased I have a daughter who was able to visit, and cared enough to do so. Mum was obviously really pleased too.

Thursday 4 January

I had a very special time on Wednesday with Margaret from the church. She says she is thinking of undertaking a distance learning theology course run by a chap from Broughton. I said I would like to find out about it too. Before she came round I had prayed in the morning that I might be able to encourage Margaret in some way, and recalled the illustration of the mosaic in Nouwen's book *Can you Drink this Cup?* We talked about living in 'community' especially the joy of being able to share with Christian brothers and sisters of all denominations.

Nouwen's illustration of the mosaic is so helpful: whether a piece is a precious stone or not, every piece matters and is noticed if it is missing. Just like a community; everyone is important. He really understood, as he worked in a community for the disabled.

I lent her the book

Friday 5 January

I had a lovely but tiring afternoon and evening in London with Marian yesterday. It was my first trip to London since my operation. At least she has work in pantomime for the rest of the month. I'm very pleased about this and the initiative she is showing.

History Boys was excellent as a stage play. I walked through Soho with Marian prior to going to the theatre. We walked through the red-light area and I pointed out to her that her grandfather had run the VD clinic for the area, when GU medicine and dermatology weren't separate specialties! Marian said how lovely it had been to visit grandma in hospital in Orpington and see signposts to the Peter Samman dermatology department, named after grandpa. I must go there when I am better, or when mum has the other knee done. It is lovely to hear how proud Marian was to see her grandfather's name commemorated!

It is very easy to walk a long way in London without realising it. I am rather pleased with what I managed, but paid the price overnight by waking up coughing again, one hour after falling asleep.

I must remember this as I plan other trips, and gradually reintroduce a pattern of work. I am not fit, and I must take it gently! I need sleep if I am going to concentrate the following day. At least I am only on call on Friday, so I can have an afternoon nap.

I have been on for the police today for Aylesbury. I was called early this morning, but it felt good getting involved again. It is an important part of my life here in Aylesbury. I must be sensible about how much I can do, and stay well, long-term.

Saturday 6 January
Disability and dying

I had a lovely chat this morning with my friend Chris, who is disabled. We talked about disability. He was happy to confirm my thought that he had never really expected to live long enough to retire. His transplanted kidney has lasted so well. He said that most of those who used to have dialysis with him are dead now. He is going to keep himself busy but, as he said, the beauty of retirement is that on days when he wakes up feeling unwell, he won't have to force himself to get up to go to work. Of course, this was something I could fully relate to, and explained that was why I was only going to undertake work with back-up by others, whilst having chemotherapy. It's good to be able to empathise with a man with such significant disability, but with such faith.

I slept well this afternoon, but had the same dream for a second time. I dreamed I was watching my death certificate being filled in. I'm not sure what to think of this, but it does not worry me. I suppose it is one of my obsessions, and what I teach the junior doctors – the importance of getting the detail absolutely correct – and I think that is what I am checking in my dream.

Sunday 7 January

I had a dreadful night's sleep with so many hot flushes. Why is it that I can sleep for two hours during the afternoon, fully clothed, under the duvet, and feel cold on waking even though the central heating is on, but at night when it is off, I get so hot in my nightshirt, that I throw off the duvet, and toss and turn?

I talked to Rachel on the phone this afternoon, after she had gone back to Manchester yesterday. She said her church service had been hard, and she had spent a lot of time in tears, one reason being that she is a long way away from me. I think I need to go up and see her sooner rather than later. I understand, she needs to keep seeing me, she was content during the Christmas holiday to come and go, but she needed regular hugs.

It is such a joy that both girls have found such caring fellowships where they live, where they can worship and receive support. At times like this I don't know how we would cope without our faith, without knowing the love of our heavenly Father. Trusting God to care for our daughters can be really hard at times, but it is wonderful to see how He works. I don't know how I would have felt if only one of them shared our faith.

I was reflecting on my 'prognosis' in church this morning. I know it is important for me to have an idea, as I didn't want to spend all my time working, only to develop an early recurrence. Time is precious; each day is important, particularly when half the time I am so tired.

Yes, time is really precious. I must also make an effort to see my mother as often as possible.

Monday 8 January

We had a good evening service yesterday. Poor Cathie reversed into my car, in the pouring rain, trying to leave quickly at the end of the service. It was minor damage only but it needed a bit of careful manoeuvring to extract her bumper from my wheel arch.

I rang her this evening. She was so much more upset than I was. I'm glad I phoned her!

Tuesday 9 January

My next chemotherapy is due tomorrow. I saw Amanda, my oncologist, this morning. I said I was feeling really well, and my blood count has recovered better on docetaxol than it did on FEC, even though we know it dropped very low at the end of December. I joked with Amanda about the website that told me not to drink alcohol whilst on docetaxol. We agreed that no explanation had been given, and that it was actually very unfair to doom your patients to eighteen weeks without alcohol, without explaining the reason! I explained I had decided to ignore the advice, but agreed that alcohol might increase the side-effects that I attribute to the dexamethasone at the start of the cycle.

I had a really good time as a day hospice patient today, doing my mosaic. Patients are starting to talk to me about many things, even evolution! One of the other patients is planning to do more crafts and join us on the craft table. It will be quite crowded, but the conversation will be good!

Lorna came in at lunchtime. She's looking very distinguished with very neat, short grey and black hair. After chemo hers doesn't seem to have come back curly, but it is so soft! Her husband Paul described her as a badger. He's right: dark in the centre and whiter over the temples.

My mood dropped after getting home this afternoon. I decided to try to have a short sleep, but thought I would check my left breast first as I am due to see Alan, my surgeon, this evening.

There is definitely a lump of some sort in my left breast, in a similar place to the tumour site in the right breast, but I no longer have the right for comparison. I am going to have to mention it tonight, but I don't want to appear neurotic. He's checked it twice before, but it is changing. I really don't want to go through any more investigations at present.

Despair and hope – a spiritual debate

What if it turns out to be another tumour?

Can I face any more surgery? Does it mean the docetaxol chemotherapy is also not working? Have I really got to start telling everyone more bad news? How can I possibly tell my daughter Rachel more bad news? There's a limit, and I am sure she has reached it. I hope it is the cyst that was seen on my first scan. I think it is time for a bit of stability. I hope tonight will be straightforward, and I will have chemo tomorrow as planned. Psalm 121 is definitely a great help at present.

> I lift up my eyes to the hills,
> From whence does my help come?
> My help comes from the Lord,
> Who made heaven and earth.
>
> He will not let your foot be moved,
> He who keeps you will not slumber.
> Behold, he who keeps Israel
> Will neither slumber nor sleep.
>
> The Lord is your keeper;
> The Lord is your shade on your right hand.
> The sun shall not smite you by day,
> Nor the moon by night.

> The Lord will keep you from all evil;
> He will keep your life.
> The Lord will keep your going out and coming in
> From this time forth and forever more.

'The Lord will keep you from all evil (or harm).' That's not just a promise for me but also for Rachel. I am suffering but I have been supported so much as well. He hasn't promised me a life without suffering, a journey without pain, but He has promised to protect me from too much harm. He has promised that for Rachel and the rest of my family as well. Mum needing surgery for another cancer – wouldn't that be too much harm for Rachel? I have had enough of breaking bad news; I don't think I can face another change of plan. She needs stability at the moment, she needs to be kept from harm and this would really harm her.

8.50 p.m.

I felt much calmer after I had battled through that this afternoon! I've never prayed like that before, reasoning with myself, and arguing with God, whilst putting my thoughts down in my journal on the computer!

God is good! I would not have coped with telling more bad news at the moment, and it would certainly have been too much for Rachel. Psalm 121 is definitely special at present!

I had a benign cyst confirmed and aspirated from my left breast, so my prayer for stability was answered. I will have the seroma fluid, which has built up below my scar, drained in two weeks time and now know I have superficial thrombophlebitis (inflammation in the veins) of right arm. Of course I do – I'm not very good at self-diagnosis – but at least it should settle with time and anti-inflammatory medication.

What should I be praying for? Blind Bartimaeus said very clearly that he wanted to be able to see (Mark 10: 51).

What do I want? Do I want healing? I want wholeness! I feel amazingly alive now; through suffering, I am growing and learning so much. It is such a precious time, and I know I am strengthening the faith of others. Ultimately, that's what is really important. But I also long to see my daughters happily married, and that needs a lot of prayer as they need boyfriends first!

Wednesday 10 January

Chemo went really smoothly today. I had a lovely chat with Andy, my GP, and June. It was so lovely to see her. If it hadn't been for her work and commitment to fundraising I wouldn't be having chemo in the comfort of that caring place. I suspect I do get preferential treatment. My specially mixed chemo arrived very quickly after being ordered!

I walked to the unit just after a downpour, and walked back with blue sky overhead. It was good to walk back as I bumped into Mary, my friend and church administrator, so she came back for a coffee. I was missed at the midweek communion. At least Mary could say where I was. It's amazing how loved I am by so many people!

I started feeling a bit sick by 3 p.m., but metoclopramide seems to work well. I hope to try to avoid the horrors of constipation this time. I slept on and off this afternoon, but managed to eat some food this evening. Hope it stays down! I think it is OK to spend time resting in bed, as my legs get so uncomfortable otherwise. I seem to be getting more and more hot flushes now, not just at night. I switched to the summer duvet, which helped a bit last night. Of course dexamethasone is making the sweats worse, so they may settle again by the weekend.

I had a really good chat with Rachel this morning, and Marian last night. It was so good to tell them some good news, and Nick too. He even won his chess match!

Reflection on brokenness (suffering)

I completed the short reflective book Life of the Beloved *today by Henri Nouwen. In it he looks at spiritual life, focusing on the bread: taken (chosen), blessed, broken and shared. My mind must be very focused at present, as I was reading the chapter about brokenness sitting in the Chiltern Hospital waiting room, knowing I had another breast lump! He talked about how we so often perceive brokenness (suffering) as a curse confirming our worthlessness. 'Children of God should pull their brokenness away from the shadow of the curse and put it under the light of blessing' (p79). That's right! 'What seemed intolerable becomes a challenge' (yes, something to be welcomed and befriended!). 'What seemed a reason for depression becomes a source of purification. What seemed punishment becomes a gentle pruning. What seemed rejection becomes a way to a deeper communion.' Of course, instinctively we want to ignore, or even deny suffering but in fact the first step to healing is to acknowledge and 'befriend' suffering. It is not masochistic to embrace suffering.*

It was a hard lesson to learn when I was trying to work at my previous practice, and I know that since then I have been trying to avoid further suffering by avoiding confrontation, for example, but after careful preparation, embracing suffering appears far more appropriate now.

I need to be careful what I say sometimes, though. When I mentioned that I was starting to enjoy being 'off sick' Alan my surgeon seemed to understand, but the radiologist thought it strange.

Nouwen points out the very personal and individual nature of our suffering (brokenness). It's not helpful to be told that hundreds of people have the same or worse problems! He talks about the suffering of the severely physically handicapped, saying that it is easier to accept the inability to speak or feed yourself, etc, than to accept the inability to be of special value to another person. Yes, I can see that. The loneliness of rejection is almost unbearable.

The final chapter talks about being broken in order to be shared with others. We become beautiful people when we can give whatever we can give: a smile, a handshake, an embrace….

He reflects that in his experience the 'happy life' is discovered through accepting our brokenness (suffering). I need to think about this further, but if he means 'wholeness', yes I believe wholeness comes through suffering, and facing up to death is very much part of this. The next book of his, Our greatest gift is all about this but it may be harder to read!

Saturday 13 January

It was my worst day today; my last dose of dexamethasone was yesterday (I divided the last dose of 8 mg into two so had 4 mg yesterday morning). I'm not sure how useful this was but my mood dipped significantly today and my bowels have been hard work. An enema helped.

Uncertainty and hope

I managed to attend a classical concert this evening. The Quartet for the End of Time by Messiaen was amazing. The programme notes were brilliant. He composed it whilst he was in a POW camp in 1941, with no idea whether he would live or if the world would come to an end. It starts with a melody of bird songs. The piece reveals his strength of faith; his understanding of the book of Revelation. The fifth movement is a cello solo reflecting Jesus as the Word, and the final movement is a violin solo reflecting the Son returning to the Father. This reminded me of the words of Jesus on the cross: 'It is finished!' I've done it! I've reached the goal; with the Father's arms outstretched to welcome him home.

Messiaen, composing that piece when he had no idea what would happen to him, has helped me. Heb. 11: 1: 'Now faith is the assurance of things hoped for, the conviction of things not seen.' I can't see the future with any certainty at present; nor could he but he had the faith to believe that, ultimately, God does know and is in control. The open arms of the Father are for us too.

Sunday 14 January

I've had another day feeling pretty lousy with constipation, tachycardia (rapid pulse), aching legs and no energy. I just wanted to spend it in bed. I managed to go to church this morning, but found it extremely difficult as my legs were restless, and it seemed a very long service. I'm afraid it was rather an ordeal. Maybe I'll remember that in three weeks' time. Foolishly, I was also on call for the Aylesbury police. It felt good going down to do some work, but I couldn't have seen a prisoner before having a nap in the afternoon. I mustn't be on call again the weekend after chemo; it doesn't work!

Symptoms this time include aching joints at night, swollen and very restless legs, tachycardia, fatigue, irritability, throat discomfort, heartburn and constipation.

Monday 15 January

Yesterday was awful. I fell asleep thinking about storing treasure in clay jars, or even baked bean cans, like I had given the girls for Christmas! (Safes that looked like baked bean cans!)

2 Cor. 3: 18–4: 18 was perfect for the moment. 'But we have this treasure in earthen vessels (clay jars), to show that the transcendent power belongs to God and not to us. We are afflicted in every way, but not crushed; perplexed but not driven to despair; persecuted, but not forsaken; struck down, but not destroyed' (v7). 'So we do not lose heart. Though our outer nature is wasting away, our inner nature is being renewed every day' (v16).

Before reading the passage I was so uncomfortable, and I had been wondering how I was going to get to sleep after a long sleep in the afternoon, and confined to bed all evening. I realised at that moment that the thought of going to sleep, without any hope of waking up to find things were better, was something I really did not want to face. I was looking at a packet of sleeping tablets by my bed. One tablet would be enough to get me off to sleep, but I could take more…. That level of despair is a new experience for me. Perhaps the verse should say 'not driven to *total* despair'. Fortunately, I knew that things would improve over the next twenty-four hours or so.

In fact my mood and energy levels improved at lunchtime today.

Reflection on my need for solitude

I tried to sleep after lunch but palpitations due to my fast pulse rate prevented this, so I lay in bed thinking about going for a walk, and thinking about the canal. I thought about the number of locks that a barge goes through to reach the top at Marsworth. It's hard work, going uphill and there are no short cuts, and it can't be done in a hurry. The route is planned and you just have to keep going.

I find walking beside the Grand Union Canal can be a very rewarding time for me. There are so many different stretches, all with their own unique features and variety of wildlife. Walking on my own gives me time to think, reflect and pray. I am aware I often think allegorically, and features of the canal often inspire me. When I began my cancer journey I stood by the canal and reflected on how far you can travel along the canal, and how long my journey would take. The Lord didn't promise an easy journey, only that he would always be with me. Just like a barge on the canal, the going is smooth and easy until you come to a lock, and then it is hard work for a while.

Being quiet and spending time alone with God enables me to listen to Him. It is often whilst standing and gazing at the 'still waters' that I feel closest to God, and most loved. He knows my love of the countryside. I can praise the Creator, and enjoy the beautiful little details with Him. My soul is restored, but it takes time and discipline. It doesn't happen in an instant.

As I failed to fall asleep I decided to go for a walk in the afternoon. I wanted to see if I could find another way to the hide at Wilstone reservoir, as the car park is a works site at present. First thought was to try Drayton Beauchamp, but the road was closed, so I needed a rethink; so I drove round to Tringford and parked by the cemetery. I thought I could find my way to the hide and took a shortcut across the field, but although I regained the footpath I could not find the path to the hide. I kept walking, promising myself I would be able to rest my legs in the hide when I reached it. I wandered further, over several stiles, until I realised I had gone far too far, and reached houses. I had walked to Drayton Beauchamp. It's a beautiful village, but a long way from where I had parked.

I didn't want to walk back over the fields, I was tired, I didn't have my mobile or any money, or a map with me and it was going to be dark in an hour. I had been very foolish, considering how ill I had been. I walked up the road passed the church and realised I had reached the Wendover branch of the Grand Union Canal, where restoration is taking place. Here was a clear path across the top of the ridge which would get me back to my car! Suddenly I could start enjoying the walk; I was no longer lost, and beside the path there was even a map telling me exactly how far I would need to walk!

The weather was beautiful. The low sun was behind me. A flock of redwings flew over. The red under their wings could be clearly seen. There was a beautiful view of the reservoir from the ridge. I would have had that view earlier, too, if I hadn't taken the shortcut! However, it was wonderful looking at it as the sun set. I walked along the canal path looking at the excavation work. I thought about the volunteers who spend their spare time digging, and concreting to restore the canal. It's not a short-term project; it is taking years. It requires commitment, dedication and perseverance. It looks ugly at present but eventually the canal will be beautiful, and it will be so good to see barges using it again; restored, rejuvenated and fully functional again. Flourishing again!

Reflecting on this, the same message comes across. No shortcuts, it's not worth it; you lose the way and miss the view. It's hard work, restoration takes a very long time and requires perseverance, but the reward is great.

Relax and enjoy each moment! When I was lost I couldn't take in my surroundings or enjoy the beauty of God's creation, but getting back on the right path meant I could make the most of the time, and the view.

Eventually, I stood beside the reservoir looking at the sunset and watched and listened to the wigeons whistling. Their pink breast feathers looked wonderful illuminated by the glow of the deep pink sunlight.

Wednesday 17 January
Thought on giving

Giving is far more than just tithing money. As long as I can keep giving to people, blessing them and restoring them in some way I will be happy. To see someone start to flourish again is a great privilege, but it doesn't necessarily have to be as part of my paid work! This is something I've been thinking about. I have had so much more time recently to sit and listen to my friends.

Even if there are times when I can't speak out loud I can still pray in silence, and enjoy fellowship with God.

Yesterday was a wonderful day!

I went to day hospice in the morning and found the mosaic-making extremely fulfilling and satisfying. And how about this: a new definition of 'joy' given me by Margaret the volunteer! It's cutting a piece of tile and finding it fits exactly into the space!

I had lunch and met up with Margaret from church at Stoke Mandeville station to go to London at 1 p.m. I realised she was excited about going, even though we only had £10 limited view seats to see *The 39 Steps*. This was Marian's Christmas present to me: cheap seats but with the hope we would be upgraded, but she hadn't expected to be working and unable to accompany me. I hadn't realised how much of an adventure it was for Margaret. She hadn't travelled to London by train for ages and was amused by my regular routine.

When we reached the theatre we were told the upper circle was closed but we would be upgraded – how sad! The man in the box office described Marian as a 'shrewd character' as he gave us £39.50 seats instead. We were just admiring our wonderful view when we were all ordered to evacuate the building (the Criterion). I felt dreadful after bringing Margaret all that way, but it was a false alarm, and it added to the atmosphere. The play was the most enjoyable thing I have seen in a long time. It was hilarious and the timing of the four actors was amazing!

We met up with Marian afterwards and walked towards Häagen-Dazs, Leicester Square, only to find our way blocked by a huge crowd waiting to see the stars arrive for a cinema premiere. A policeman let us through and we found the ice cream restaurant nearly empty. (I had expected to have to queue outside for at least ten minutes.) God is good – every little detail of the day worked perfectly, and Margaret went on up to Camden to celebrate her daughter's birthday with her to round off the evening.

Medical review

Yes I probably overdid it! But I didn't fall asleep in the train on the way home!

I fell asleep quite early and quickly, but woke about 2.30 a.m. and was awake until after 4 a.m. The symptoms during the night included dyspepsia, in spite of increasing lansoprazole to 30 mg twice daily, and mildly aching joints, but I didn't want to take ibuprofen in the middle of the night when I had only just relieved my dyspepsia with gaviscon! However my main problem is burning fingertips. I had noticed that during the last cycle, but it was transient. A peripheral neuropathy is a side-effect of docetaxol. It returned yesterday and now it is making writing, fine movements and typing more difficult. I still managed to do my mosaic so I shouldn't fuss!

Nick and I both woke up early. It was so lovely just to snuggle up and relax in bed, and read the newspaper together without rushing around, especially as it's midweek. It is very important not to neglect having time together at the moment.

This afternoon I had a special treat, I went to day hospice and a lady from Eaton-Bray was demonstrating two owls – a barn owl and a tawny. She allowed us to handle the tawny and flew the barn owl around day hospice! It was so lovely to see the joy on the faces of the patients. Fortunately, I remembered my camera, so I will be able to give photos to the patients and we may be able to do a display. That's right, as I thought at the beginning of the day, 'as long as I can keep giving....'

Friday 19 January
Ethical reflection

I fell asleep last night reflecting on what constitutes 'harm', thinking spiritually and ethically – 'medical harm'. My mind is definitely doing strange things at the moment. I had a very bizarre but significant dream. I dreamed that someone was trying to poison me by throwing poison-tipped needles at me. I then lay there waiting for the poison to take effect – waiting to die and wondering why it wasn't happening.

I think I may have had this dream before – it is vaguely familiar, but this is the third in a series of dreams relating to my cancer, the others being the horrors of chest wall recurrence of the cancer, and making sure my death certificate is written out correctly!

I talked about my symptoms over the weekend at the hospice and my concern at my thoughts of despair. What would I have thought about if I hadn't had the medical knowledge that the symptoms would resolve? That level of agitation is so unpleasant. I didn't know how to get comfortable. I was in and out of bed, up and downstairs. I tried to sit on the settee for a few minutes but then went back to bed. I kept looking at the time and hardly any time had gone by. Was it time to go to sleep yet? Would I get to sleep? And then thinking if it doesn't get any better, would I want to go through another day like that?

I've watched so many patients become agitated, and listened to families talking about their loved one constantly asking what the time is, and struggling to sit for more than a few minutes in one place – so restless. I also remember the weekend more than a decade ago when I was so stressed about what would happen at work on Monday – would I be able to cope? Would the bullying and hateful behaviour on the part of both my practice manager and her husband be even worse? When would it stop? I couldn't concentrate on anything, nor could I settle. A minute felt like an hour.

It is difficult being both a doctor and a patient. Would I have associated the symptoms with side-effects of treatment if I were just a lay person? Would I have had the assurance I needed to persevere if I weren't a professional? How much should we warn patients about potential side-effects but without putting them off the treatment? This, of course is a recurrent problem in general practice. You can spend time with patients in distress, with significant depression. You feel you have managed to overcome their fears of inadequacy about not being able to 'snap out of it', and having to 'give in to the problem'. You persuade them that medication may be able to help them over a few weeks, only to find on follow-up that they haven't started on treatment because they've read the drug information leaflet and fear an obscure side-effect, or are worried about an irrelevant drug interaction. I know it is important to mention possible agitation with some medication in depression, but tend to play it down. Now that I have experienced this level of agitation with dexamethasone, maybe I won't be so dismissive. If despair plus agitation can produce even transient suicidal thoughts, this has to be taken seriously. At least if the patient starts on medication for depression you are at last providing them with some hope for the future. It is the lack of hope during suffering which is so damaging. Giving hope is one of the most therapeutic things we can do. During the consultation where there is total despair, to offer some consolation is to rekindle hope. Luke 22: 43 tells us that at the moment of Jesus's greatest distress and sorrow, in the garden of Gethsemane, he was ministered to by an angel and strengthened so he approached the soldiers boldly and calmly. During a consultation, even in despair it is often possible to create a lighter moment and laughter. That special moment, a moment of joy, offers a glimmer of hope. It really is rewarding when the patient reaches the door and turns saying: 'Thank you, I feel better already.' No medication has been taken but the patient has been listened to, respected, and somehow found hope again. Maybe it is because they know help is available, but maybe it was a moment of laughter that illuminated the darkness.

How can we balance the benefits of our therapies without causing harm, either by failing to warn of serious – if unlikely – side-effects, or by putting the patient off and thus destroying that glimmer of hope? How can we ensure we keep our patients safe without causing harm by making them so anxious about the side-effects they don't start the treatment?

This is, of course, most important when the alternative to therapy is a certain but lingering death from metastatic cancer. On the other hand there is a point, especially with chemotherapy, where the desire to keep hope alive by offering another course may in fact cause more harm than good and increase the patient's suffering at the end of life; improving symptom control would in fact be a better option.

The answer for me may be to explain how I felt but trying to make light of it, if the concern is transient agitation, by emphasising that it will be short-lived.

In medical ethics casuistry has had a chequered history, but in medicine we often learn from cases, and some cases are so significant that they modify practice (paradigm cases) in the same way as legal cases can modify common law – something, as a police surgeon, I am very familiar with.

Will my practice change as a result of my experience? Am I a paradigm case?

Saturday 20 January

We travelled down to Hever yesterday after seeing my mother. She is amazing: three weeks after a total knee replacement she leaps out of a chair and moves very swiftly across the room without any walking aid.

We had a lovely walk through Bedgebury Pinetum this morning; not too windy, warm and sunny and beautiful blue sky. We visited our friends Robin and Helen this afternoon. I used to work with Helen in general practice in Maidstone, and we trained together. It was a lovely drive through the Weald of Kent looking at oast houses and orchards. I had forgotten how well Kent fits the title the 'Garden of England'.

Sunday 21 January

Nick's birthday!

It was another lovely sunny day. We went back to Vinters Park, Maidstone – where we used to live – to worship with Verity Christian Fellowship, the new Vinters Christian community that we had helped set up about eighteen years ago. I felt so 'at home' worshipping again in the community centre. It was so encouraging to see Gerry leading the worship and to stand and sing with Chris. They prayed specifically for me. The drummer prayed and referred to psalm 40:

> *I waited patiently for the Lord,*
> *He inclined to me and heard my cry.*
> *He drew me up from the desolate pit,*
> *Out of the miry bog,*

And set my feet upon a rock,
Making my steps secure.
He put a new song in my mouth,
A song of praise to our God.
Many will see and fear, and put their trust in the Lord.

Many will… put their trust in the Lord, is my prayer.

Chris introduced me to a friend who had breast cancer seven years ago and went through chemo. I recognised her but couldn't think why. She then mentioned she had been a GP receptionist, and I realised she had worked with Helen and me!

Monday 22 January

We travelled back from Kent today. We tried to find somewhere open to visit but really struggled. Eventually, we spent some time at Waltham Abbey. It was good to reflect on the fact that people have worshipped there for more than 1,000 years – possibly since AD 600. King Harold (killed at battle of Hastings) founded the present building (a bit remains). When Henry VIII dissolved the monasteries, Thomas Tallis was the organist. It is lovely to think that the wonderful piece that has inspired the beautiful arrangement by Vaughan Williams was probably first heard there.

Very caring people keep asking me how I am, and really want to know.

Reflecting, on the way home today, I decided to list the good and the bad times. It is so easy to focus on the moment and the way I am feeling at the time. I shouldn't just focus on the bad days, to gain sympathy, but also highlight the blessings. It would be good to put the blessings into succinct and everyday language.

So let's try weighing up the advantages and disadvantages, the good from the bad, the blessings from the struggles. That's a very utilitarian approach, even though I cannot adhere to the utilitarian approach to decision-making – maximising happiness and minimising pain – as I sincerely believe that by always trying to avoid suffering you can miss real blessing. By listing the benefits and the problems encountered through the suffering caused by my cancer, this should become clear. By accepting the challenge it is becoming a great time of cleansing, healing and refreshment. Nick has been saying it has been good as we have been able to spend more time together. Initially, I was amused as we may be in the same house but often in different rooms, but we have more meals together and more times of relaxation, when we enjoy watching or listening to the same thing.

Advantages:
- Time with the family.
- Having time for friends.
- New and deeper relationships.
- Being able to support and encourage friends in their troubles, without feeling exhausted by work commitments.
- Realising how much I am loved!
- All the wonderful cards from everyone.
- Realising how much I am valued by patients.
- Healing psychological hurts; reflecting on the therapeutic nature of laughter.
- Feeling well enough, and having sufficient time, to reflect on the difficult days so I can learn from them and help others.
- Time to reflect and to pray.

- *Time for walking, especially by the canal. Time for growth – I am no longer too busy to learn from my experiences.*
- *Being able to spend time reflecting without sleep deprivation. In the last couple of years my main reflective times have been either on holiday, or when driving to and from Wycombe, in the middle of the night; great times of reflection, but constantly stressed by the fear of not coping with work the next day, due to sleep deprivation.*
- *Learning from my symptoms to encourage greater openness in day hospice etc.*
- *Having time off from work (refreshment).*
- *Being able to be creative through writing, digital photography and making my mosaic – having time to explore new skills, and enhancing those I already had.*
- *A wonderful selection of hats!*

Disadvantages:
- *Struggling with symptoms:*
    - *Constipation*
    - *Fluctuating mood*
    - *Agitation and restlessness (transient)*
    - *Hot flushes*
    - *Loss of hair.*
- *Not being able to work (financially).*
- *Not being able to work (deskilling and getting out of date).*
- *Difficult routine with so much medication.*
- *Knowing I will go through all the side-effects again and again.*
- *Seeing the family struggling.*

Tuesday 23 January

It was cold during the night. My head was particularly cold. I eventually realised what the problem was and put my woolly hat on and then settled.

I woke up early thinking I would love a cup of coffee and then remembered I should take my lansoprazole first, and leave a gap before drinking any milk as it affects the absorption of the drug. I took the medication and promptly went back to sleep, waking at 8.30 a.m.

That was OK today as I didn't need to leave the house to go to day hospice until around 10.30 a.m., but in two weeks time I'm meant to be going back to work there and need to be there by 8.45 a.m. at the latest. I managed well today without an afternoon nap but I'm not sure what it will be like when I work, as well as attending day hospice to be creative with the patients doing my mosaic.

I do feel much more alive today. A few aches and pains appeared only after concentrating hard at the surgery, inputting data in the afternoon. My tired body told me when to stop and go home, and I listened!

I had a good chat with Rachel my practice manager. It is time to discuss with my partners what I find so easy to talk to Rachel about: my future in the practice and her vision for the practice overall. It was really encouraging to talk to Rachel like this and realise how important the future of the practice is to her. She has a real vision. It is fantastic to think that she is thinking so long-term – in fact, thinking that she will remain in the practice long after we have all left! I must tell her how encouraged I was, when I next see her, and push for some of her plans to be realised.

For the first time, today I could see that my illness could be used creatively to enhance and develop the practice. I had been so worried about discussing the future with my partners, but now Rachel has given me hope there. I wonder if Rachel would have thought so constructively about it if I hadn't been off sick.

I know the Lord's timing is always perfect but sometimes it is hard to see the bigger picture. If we had all been well we would have carried on regardless with the same routine; with me struggling to cope with the amount of work and lack of sleep, especially during holiday times; with both partners and fellow police surgeons away, needing cover; but this would have been foolish. My illness is an opportunity for reappraisal.

Wednesday 24 January

I woke up at 3.30 a.m. and thought it was far too light outside, but dismissed the idea of snow. I woke again at 6.40 a.m. and realised how quiet it was outside; there really was snow on the ground. Everything looked white.

It was a really special day today. I took the photos into day hospice, for the patients I had photographed I had taken a week ago with the barn and tawny owls. They loved them.

I went to London in the afternoon. I had arranged an appointment at Nicola Jane, the mastectomy wear shop between Angel and the Barbican. It was a wonderfully professional service and care; the assistant was so encouraging and sensitive. I am so glad I went there so I could try different bras and prostheses. I now feel so good with a proper well-fitted prosthesis. The timing of my appointment with Alan yesterday evening, to have my seroma drained and my trip to London today, was perfect. I couldn't be fitted properly if I still had fluid under the scar.

I walked across the Millennium Bridge from St Paul's to the Tate Modern as the sun began to set. I was very tempted just to stay on the bridge and watch the sunset, but I'm glad I went into the gallery. I found a few lovely pictures to look at: a Monet of water lilies and a fantastic seascape painted by a Danish artist. It was a menacing sky and rough sea – a storm. It's lovely there to be able to sit in the middle of the room, and spend time reflecting on the pictures.

When I woke this morning, I started thinking about the last art gallery I had been to – the Lowry at Salford Quays. I remembered one picture in particular: a picture he had painted after the death of his mother. It is a picture of the sea but not a stormy, colourful seascape but just grey/white waves, the horizon and a grey sky above. I was struck at the time the length of time it must have taken to build up the texture of the waves – the detail was amazing – but what struck me on waking today was how long he had spent staring at the sea. Some of his paintings had a ship in them but this had nothing; nothing on the horizon, nothing but shades of grey. He was profoundly depressed. It is a picture of despair with no hope for the future – nothing on the horizon.

I had a glimpse of what that can feel like two weekends ago after my chemo, and I'm beginning to grow anxious about the next lot in a week's time – can I avoid the same awful experience? However, my picture, although grey, would have had something else in it – a boat or perhaps a lighthouse, as even in the bleakest moments, I still have hope.

Thursday 25 January

I went to Apothecaries' Hall yesterday evening. It was lovely to see Kim, the registrar, and some old friends from the philosophy course, especially Don and Trent. They all recognised me with no hair but wearing a hat. I had forgotten how posh the occasion would be. I wasn't really dressed smartly enough, but of course I was wearing my new bra and brand new prosthesis and felt great!

I am so glad Trent got a distinction in the philosophy exam, and the prize. I didn't know there was a prize and certainly wasn't expecting it to be awarded to him last night. I'm so glad I made the effort to go so I could be there to celebrate with him, and congratulate him! He is such an intelligent young man, but so unassuming.

Friday 26 January

We had a staff lunch in day hospice. I proudly showed off my new shape! I have never done this before, even when I was younger. Having a properly fitted bra and a perfectly symmetrical prosthesis has done wonders for my self-esteem! In the past I was far too busy to even check if I looked symmetrical: I just wore shapeless sweatshirts and thick jumpers, and didn't worry. Now I only have one real breast I want to wear clothes that make me feel more feminine, and now I can! Jane, our community specialist palliative care nurse, was so impressed she asked for the name of the shop for her other clients. She also said that it looked as if I had had a 'boob job' rather than a mastectomy. At present I am certainly not thinking of reconstruction surgery – I am happy with what I have now. It was well worth the time and money to be properly fitted. I must write to the company to let them know.

Monday 29 January

I went into the surgery and spent four hours there putting data onto the computer and had a meeting with my partners and practice manager. I agreed that it was important to spell out my terms, what I want to do in the future, and how much I think I will be able to do. I emphasised my prognosis and my desire to have more time to do the things I really want to do, and I don't want to have to say to the girls: 'I'm working so I can't see your performance.'

Reflection on a portrait of despair

I reflected on yesterday evening's informal service at church. I wanted to ask for prayer for next weekend which may well be awful, if the pattern is the same as my last chemo cycle. I hadn't been sure whether I should say anything but had planned to refer to psalm 42. When Roger began the service by reciting psalm 42 I realised it was appropriate to say something.

> As a hart longs for flowing streams,
> So longs my soul for thee, O God.
> My soul thirsts for God, for the living God.
> When shall I come and behold the face of God?
> My tears have been my food day and night,
> While men say to me continually,
> 'Where is your God?'
> These things I remember, as I pour out my soul:

How I went with the throng,
And led them in procession to the house of God,
With glad shouts and songs of thanksgiving,
A multitude keeping festival.

Why are you cast down, O my soul,
And why are you disquieted within me?
Hope in God;
For I shall again praise him,
My help and my God.

'Hope and lack of hope' were the key points and that was exactly the theme of the sermon, as well and the chosen songs for worship. I wanted to illustrate my feeling of despair so people could understand. I talked about the portrait of the sea painted by Lowry we had seen before Christmas – an amazing picture, which I could have stared at for hours, as Lowry had stared at the sea. A portrait of sea and sky with nothing on the horizon, painted after his mother died when he was depressed and lonely. For me it was a portrait of despair: nothing to cling onto, nothing on the horizon, no hope.

I explained how bad I had felt. I was low in mood but also agitated and restless. I was watching the clock. I do not know what I would have done without hope, without the knowledge that it was temporary, and God is in control.

I asked for prayer (and received it) that either it would not be as bad, or I would remember psalm 42: 'Why are you cast down, O my soul, and why are you disquieted within me? Hope in God; for I shall again praise him, my help and my God.'

People prayed for me, and then we continued in prayer for others who shared similar feelings, but had been unable to verbalise them in the way I had. It was a very moving time.

After the service Roger thanked me. I felt very humble; what I had said really did seem to have enhanced the service, although I had no idea what had been planned. Roger said that it had been 'prophetic', which was rather overwhelming. However, I had woken up with a picture in my mind and I had reflected on its meaning and applied it to my situation, and what I had said had spoken to other people. There was a message from God for other people in what I had said, and that, in a nutshell, is a simple definition of prophecy.

It's also the way I communicate difficult ideas both at home and in general practice. If I am trying to explain something to a patient, I find it easier to apply the problem to myself and say 'this is how I manage', rather than 'you should do this'. Now, on two occasions in church, people have listened to my prayer request, and then reflected and applied it to themselves. The Lord isn't just caring for me in this, but caring and ministering to others in the church through me, even though I am not doing my daytime job at present. But He hasn't taken me beyond my comfort zone; only to the limits.

I spoke to my daughter Rachel on the phone. She loved the picture of the sea by Lowry when she went to the exhibition just over a week ago, with Marian. I must ask Marian what she thought of it too.

Tuesday 30 January

I had a really bad night. I had noticed that I had had increased chest pain and a sore throat during the day, but woke up twice with severe chest pain which eventually settled with gaviscon, and increasing the number of pillows. This had come on in spite of taking 60 mg lansoprazole daily. This alarmed me as I had to restart dexamethasone today which might make it even worse.

At times like this I need to look at Psalms. I looked at psalm 34. Should I read it again tomorrow? I discussed my symptoms with Amanda, my oncologist, in clinic, but we agreed I would be continuing with the same dose of chemo.

I went on to day hospice and made great progress with my mosaic. After lunch I went to the hospice communion service, and then came home. David the chaplain read psalm 139, emphasising in prayer (v23): 'Search me, O God and know my heart; test me and know my anxious thoughts' (New international version). This seemed so appropriate as there were four of us plus David. Of course, as cancer patients, we all have anxious thoughts.

Wednesday 31 January

Chemo today (second dose of docetaxol). It went well. I had a good laugh and chat with a lady who is just starting herceptin. She needs a dose every three weeks for the next year. I do hope she doesn't get too many side-effects. What a long haul!

I had a lovely chat with June and Phyllis. Phyllis has just started as a volunteer and today was her first time working on a Wednesday. It was so good to have her making me tea and coffee and looking after my non-medical needs. I am so glad she will be there for me, and I know she is so pleased to be there too. She seems to have found a special place to serve after all those months that Allan had treatment there, and we cared for him as he was dying.

It was good to talk. My fellow patient is now thinking of reconstructive surgery, eighteen months after mastectomy. She said she certainly wasn't thinking about reconstruction during her chemo, but has struggled with prostheses following a bad reaction to her radiotherapy. I am keeping an open mind; it was good to chat – I hope she appreciated it too!

Spiritual reflection

I'm beginning to realise how useful it is to put down my thoughts like this. I keep on having new ideas, inspired thoughts, or at least they are new to me! I believe these thoughts are inspired by God in a way that suits my personality, and within my comfort zone, in the way I have learnt to reflect, in the way I have learnt to counsel and guide people through years of general practice. I have been taught to reason and reflect, much more so over the last couple of years. I have a greater understanding of God and I understand myself and others better. I have greater insight but I'm slow; I can't come up with quick answers! I became very aware of that on the philosophy course when I used to think of the best answers on the train going home! Surely it is better to spend time thinking something through? God understands; he made me as I am and has trained me. We are all unique; he works through people in different ways but knows what's best for each of us. Ever since I became a Christian, illustrations from nature have spoken to me at times very profoundly, even cutting bracken in a bird reserve at the age of seventeen spoke of cleansing.

He has just spoken to me much more profoundly in recent months. I've had time to listen, time to reflect, but also I've wanted to listen and I've been willing to listen. I have also been willing to, and taken the opportunity to tell others. It has become a real blessing. I must not become complacent or arrogant. At least exploration of this gift and reflection on its nature has come through suffering. What a gift suffering is when it is accepted and even welcomed!

I know I have an ability to verbalise and express how I feel without embarrassment. Sometimes it must be hard for the listener and I must be sensitive, but I think it is a gift. A willingness to be open and honest, whilst acknowledging we all have some secrets too painful to share, makes you vulnerable. However, the more open you are the more you can help and encourage others, and the closer the community grows, and how much more precious! No secrets are hidden from God. The Trinity is the great model of community in loving relationship. In Heaven we will have no secrets, nothing to hide. The Christian community is a taste of the Kingdom of God, and it is good.

Psalm 34: 8: 'O taste and see that the Lord is good! Happy is the man who takes refuge in Him!'

February 2007

Thursday 1 February
Medical review

I woke up (very late!) post-chemo, not feeling sick and had the courage, thinking so many have been praying about it, not to take the strong anti-emetic, granesetron. I just took metoclopramide which I know doesn't cause constipation. I had also taken one sachet of movicol yesterday, and took another sachet in the morning, to try to overcome the dreadful effects of severe constipation.

Marian arrived at 11.20 a.m. We had a wonderful time chatting about all her work and the Lowry and football paintings we have all seen.

We went to the Oaks Christian coffee and book shop. This was great as she could do some advertising, and chat to Jan who is being so supportive of both my girls. John from church was there too, before going off to Russia next week. We chatted about his healing ministry. I'm so glad he saw me looking pretty good post-chemo, after he had prayed for me on Sunday.

We had a short introduction to my locally based theology course in the afternoon. That's rather exciting, but I will need to keep up with the workload when I can concentrate!

Marian met her old school friend Leigh in the evening – he brought me flowers!

Friday 2 February

I slept in again – until 9.20 a.m.!

I had a very quiet day, and my mood was subdued (still on dexamethasone but only 4 mg today, with 2 mg on Saturday and 2 mg on Sunday, to tail them off). I had a spontaneous bowel motion – only a little uncomfortable – what a joy! Well that's another new definition of joy!

I became irritable after supper. My legs were aching and I was unable to get comfortable, so I took myself up to bed shortly after 8 p.m. and watched *The Italian Job* – the original – on my computer in bed. That was an excellent piece of distraction and escapism. I felt a lot better by 10 p.m., and had a glass of madeira, which I could taste and enjoy. Eventually I settled, after 11 p.m., after listening to a CD.

Saturday 3 February

I woke up this morning to find we had a power cut. Fortunately, power was restored before I wanted a shower. It was a very frosty night and an amazingly cloudless sky most of the day. Fantastic weather!

I went to our church coffee morning. I had a great chat with my friend Chris, joking about the time that he came to our house and promptly removed his below-knee prosthesis. I explained I wasn't planning to do the same. He laughed and laughed. We also talked about sexuality and disability in relation to teenagers in a hospice environment as it has been in the news.

Chris retired last month; he's a bit older than me. We talked about early retirement. He looks so relaxed! As he said, his transplanted kidney won't last forever, and he's being realistic. We discussed the statistic I had been given of approximately 60 per cent chance of me reaching sixty.

I was aware that many people have been praying for me and because the weather was so amazing, I decided to go to College Lake for a walk and look at the ducks, immediately after lunch. I arrived at about 1.15 p.m. and thought I would have plenty of time; actually, I walked all the way round in glorious sunshine, and left just before the gates closed at 4 p.m.

So many robins were singing and the catkins were in full bloom. I took some lovely photos including a row of cormorants with wings outstretched and teal in perfect sunlight. I saw a fieldfare quite close, plus redwings and a bullfinch. The highlight of the walk was a fantastic view of four male goldeneyes and one female, even better through another visitor's telescope.

I had a good chat with an older man with a limp. He advised me to buy a monopod (instead of a tripod) to steady the camera or scope with one hand but which would also be useful as a discreet walking stick – what an excellent idea. I had told him I wasn't very well. I slipped on the path once and noticed I can be unsteady.

I walked the two-mile walk around the reserve. There is a steep climb up a field to the top track. They've placed an old bus shelter there so people can rest. As I sat down on the bench the view was wonderful and the weather beautiful. I am finding climbing quite hard and my heart was racing. I thought to myself that if I had to, I would be more than happy to die looking at the view, but of course I walked on to the next hide!

I disturbed a hibernating bat in the hide. I looked at the whistling wigeon and one lonely shelduck visible from that hide but I was looking directly into the sun so visibility was poor.

Other birds seen: golden plover and lapwings, herons, pochard, gadwall, shoveler, coots and moorhens, mallard, etc. This was a fantastic day and so much better than my previous post-chemo weekend experience.

England even won the rugby!

Monday 5 February

What an amazing day yesterday was. I am overwhelmed by the love and care everyone is showing me. I have never felt so excited about going to church before. I just want to be with my family – my church family – to show them that prayer works!

I am also amazed by the wonderful love shown to Rachel yesterday. Her friend Esther's parents invited her to Sunday dinner, telling Esther to drive her to Rochdale for the meal at their house. They have being praying for me in their fellowship group, even though they have never met me. They've been praying for me because Rachel is a friend of both their son and daughter, but they hadn't even met her. They decided to invite her to dinner so they could get to know her. Roast beef and Yorkshire pudding as well!

Reflection on answered prayer

I can't remember our church ever feeling so much like a close family as it does at the moment. Margaret, preaching yesterday evening, was talking about loneliness, hurts and a time twenty years ago when she felt abandoned by God. I've not heard her speak in public like that before. She suddenly felt close to God again as she was driving past the police station singing psalm 42, (as you do!). Psalm 42 is so meaningful at the moment: 'Why are you cast down O my soul... I shall again praise him, my help and my God.' Her sermon was actually about faith, and holding on to faith.

A week last Sunday, at the evening service, I had said that it would be a miracle if I were in church in the evening the following Sunday, which was yesterday, as I had had such a rough time with my chemo side-effects the previous cycle. I didn't want to go to church in the evening if to do so would be a lie, and I really wasn't well enough. But I did want to go if we could celebrate!

Earlier in the week, pre-chemo, I had been reading psalm 34. I prayed that if this were a promise that I would be better this time, then I would read it at the beginning of the service on Sunday evening.

> I will bless the Lord at all times;
>   his praise shall continually be in my mouth.
> My soul makes its boast in the Lord;
>   let the afflicted hear and be glad.
> O magnify the lord with me,
>   and let us exalt his name together!
>
> I sought the Lord, and he answered me,
>   and delivered me from all my fears.

Look to him, and be radiant;
So your faces shall never be ashamed.
This poor man cried, and the Lord heard him;
and saved him out of all his troubles.
The angel of the Lord encamps around those who fear him,
and delivers them.
O taste and see that the Lord is good!
Happy is the man who takes refuge in him!

For 'poor man' read 'poor woman', if you like, but I am staggered by how meaningful and true that was for me last night, particularly the deliverance from fear. That was what was really getting to me – the fear of going through the same awful time, and knowing that could be repeated again and again and again.

I am overwhelmed by how many people have been praying – I certainly don't deserve that – and so systematically as well, during the day. Mary said she had been having sleepless nights as well, yet I went for a fantastic walk round College Lake on Saturday, and got really carried away in the worship on Sunday. I know others found that great too, though!

What's more, I know people are still praying.

Of course, I still have aches and pains, and sleep is intermittent, but the prayer I asked for last Sunday was from psalm 42 to 'hope in God; for I shall again praise him, my help (saviour) and my God'. I asked that I would keep holding on to hope in God even in despair, knowing I would again be able to praise. Instead, I was standing in church full of praise and having the time of my life! Oh, how I love singing!

I think I was rather high! In fact, I know I laughed and joked a bit when I was speaking, which was amazing. I think I shocked people last week as it is so unlike me to talk of having such a low mood, but by *being honest and verbalising inner fears, people have been drawn closer. In the family there are good and bad times; emotions, anger, fears and inadequacies are clearly seen. I know the church family should be this sort of close community as well, where we don't feel ashamed to admit our weaknesses, exposing our fears to our friends. It's crazy to pretend that everything is wonderful, and nothing ever goes wrong. We are learning to carry each other's burdens. How can we do so if we aren't prepared to admit them?*

Tuesday 6 February
My first day back at work at the hospice

It was a frosty but absolutely beautiful morning. I would have missed that if I hadn't had to go to work, so that was a real bonus!

I am glad I went back today to work during the morning, but also glad I insisted that I also attend day hospice in the afternoon, for my art therapy (my mosaic). The patients didn't seem to get confused by my changing roles, and it certainly ensures I see the day hospice patients regularly.

Medical review

During my ward round, one of the in-patients noticed I was wearing a hat, and realised the answer to her own question as she asked me why. This lady, who has had such complex needs for a very long time, cried because I have cancer.

I discussed constipation with Jane, our pharmacist, and then with one of the patients. I realised I was being much more emphatic about the horrors of constipation and the need to prevent it. I also found myself saying to another patient, how important it is to get a balance between the benefits and side-effects of the drugs we use. I hope she benefits from my recent experience of drug side-effects!

It was Lorna's first day back as well. She looked so well. Her hair has grown back so nicely post-chemo. I hope mine does too.

I am aware that today was the first day I have spent time writing in notes, or writing much at all, and this has made me aware of my mild peripheral neuropathy. I hope I will be able to put a drip up on the patient they want me to sort out on Thursday. When I am typing I am aware of fingertip pain, and some clumsiness. My fingertips and toes do burn at night.

I am also struggling again with mucocytis (a term used to describe the nasty effects chemo can have on the gut). Quite a lot of my gut seems to be affected this time. It does seem to be getting worse. I also have chest pain on and off, plus an unpleasant taste in my mouth, which is sore in places, but not ulcerated. My lips are sore. Grapefruit and gooseberry and rhubarb yogurt taste nice, so do white wine and tea, but coffee has to be very weak, and red wine would be a complete waste of money.

My bowels are also affected. After my awful constipation last cycle, I was aware of a degree of urgency, but thought this might have been due to overstimulation with laxatives. This is almost certainly, in fact, a consequence of the chemo, as I have the same problem this time. I would far rather be loose than impacted!

My scalp feels tender again this evening. I wonder if the rest of my hair is about to fall out.

I'm also still getting sufficient aches and pains over my chest wall, and in my legs, to make sleep quite difficult without ibuprofen. But I have managed to sleep over the last two nights quite well, without a sleeping tablet.

After finishing at the hospice today I had a rest. I am not sure if I slept or not, but I will try to rest completely for an hour in the afternoon, and if I sleep, then that's fine!

Wednesday 7 February

We had a very heavy frost over night, but bright sunshine and a clear sky in the morning. Unfortunately, we had another power cut at 8 a.m., but power came back on at 8.45 a.m.

Margaret, from church came round for a chat and coffee just after 10 a.m. She arrived very excited and asked if I had looked outside. 'God's showering us with gold glitter!'

It was an amazing phenomenon, something neither of us had ever seen before. Minute ice crystals in the air, moving around, and sparkling in the bright sun, looked like golden glitter falling to earth. It was so beautiful. I captured it on camera, and watched it for up to an hour, until it disappeared.

I didn't have a rest this afternoon. After tea, I suddenly had abdominal discomfort and needed to go to bed for a bit.

Thursday 8 February

I woke up to snow. I managed to walk to the hospice, but that was the limit of my exercise tolerance. At least I got to work and enjoyed working. Of course I then needed to walk back again!

Friday 9 February

I spent time at the surgery but I was also on call for the police at Aylesbury. I saw two prisoners in the afternoon, and then went shopping. I found this pretty tiring. At 6.40 p.m. I had to pick up Rachel from Princes Risborough station, and take her over to Amersham. I found my right arm was aching on the way home. I realised that this was the furthest I had driven since my operation, and realised this is still quite limiting.

Saturday 10 February
Great day, but very tiring

I caught the train from Stoke Mandeville without realising I would have to travel by bus to Beaconsfield, due to engineering works. Unfortunately, we then sat outside Marylebone for fifteen minutes. I was going to a history of medicine lecture. I arrived late for the lecture, but it was fascinating. The talk was on ancient Egyptian medicine. Remedies included a treatment for migraine: hitting the patient over the head with a dead fish!

I had a good chat with Don, my philosophy and medical ethics tutor. He said that whilst discussing the Mental Capacity Act with a hospital ethics committee, rather than saying 'lasting power of attorney' he had accidentally said 'lasting power of eternity', which struck me as particularly beautiful!

I caught the train to Clapham Junction to see Marian's new flat. It is really nice and she has decorated her room very well. I asked her to have a look at the notes I had been typing up, about my traumatic time at the practice I worked in, when she was at middle school. She knew things had been difficult, but had been far too young at the time to be told the full story. She was horrified at the conversations that had taken place.

We went to an excellent Thai restaurant on the main road. Marian's mood was a bit low, and she was worried about learning her lines. She eventually attributed her low mood to seeing the *Sea Gull* the night before – good but depressing.

Reflection on drug side-effects

I picked up the Guardian *on the train back to Victoria. I was very disturbed by the report on an inquest into the death of a sixteen-year-old boy. He had just been discharged from hospital following brain surgery to remove a brain tumour. Within forty-eight hours of his discharge, his mood had become so low that he jumped in front of a car. The death was attributed to mood swings caused by dexamethasone. I know exactly how he felt. His parents said they hadn't been warned. I really think we need to be more open about the effects on mood. Of course, in palliative care we use it to elevate mood, and tail it off very carefully, but during chemo and post-neurosurgery the dose can be dropped from 16 mg to zero more quickly. I must start discussing this with my colleagues.*

Monday 12 February

I took Rachel to Princes Risborough to meet her friend Jenny, and catch a train back to Manchester. My mood dropped after I dropped her off and I cried on the way home. I cried several times during the day, and spent quite a lot of time thinking about the lad who died following brain surgery. I must talk this through with my colleagues tomorrow.

I reflected on why my mood has dropped today. Is it still due to withdrawing from dexamethasone, but rather more slowly this time, or has it been caused by Rachel and me going to see the film *Notes on a Scandal* yesterday evening? Judi Dench's character was so reminiscent of the behaviour of Mrs C towards me, when she was my practice manager, that it stirred up some difficult memories. These memories were of her overwhelming desire for friendship, and control, followed by such hatred towards me when I disagreed with her, that she screamed and she threw things at me before I left the practice.

I discussed this with Marian on the phone this evening. She said 'Mum you are *so* not over it yet!'

Tuesday 13 February

I got to work on time, and spent the morning at the hospice with the new junior doctor.

My mood is still quite labile. I had a good chat with another colleague who feels the mood problems with dexamethasone should be better highlighted, and feels sometimes the dose can be lowered too fast.

I discussed the situation with Lorna as well. She said she spent a lot of time crying whilst on chemo. I am sure this was not just because of dexamethasone, but it may well have contributed.

I had my seroma drained again today – only 55 ml this time, but if I hadn't gone today I would have had to wait three weeks. I can't risk infection having the seroma drained whilst my white cell count is low.

Wednesday 14 February
Medical reflection

Some days I don't really have time for reflection, and learning from my experience, but today I have something to mull over. Elaine, an older lady at our church, has just found out she has breast cancer, following recall after a mammogram. How do I talk to her? I want to support her but am I ready emotionally to do this, for a friend? Her prognosis, as far as the cancer is concerned, is likely to be better than mine; she may just need a lumpectomy and radiotherapy, so she is better off than me. However, she is not a healthcare professional and she will need support, and psychologically it will be hard for her. She won't find surgery easy and the whole process takes so much time and effort... I must phone her, to encourage and support her.

I left a message on Elaine's answer machine in the afternoon.

Elaine then phoned in the evening sounding quite optimistic and more concerned about Gordon, her husband, than herself.

The father of Jay Milne, the sixteen-year-old whose death was attributed to dexamethasone, was 'live' on the Today programme on Radio 4 this morning, talking about his son's death and their lack of awareness that dexamethasone could affect mood. He said Jay had started dexamethasone ten days before surgery and was on it six days after. He explained that he had been given it for acute headache and vomiting, and acknowledged that the drug is very beneficial, as it reduces swelling due to bruising after surgery. He said the operation was a base-of-skull operation, so he had been told it would not have caused the psychological problems.

He said that when Jay came home he didn't recognise his son in his actions. He added that a quiet word with them would have prevented this. He said he wanted a protocol produced to warn people.

Thursday 15 February

I worked at the hospice this morning. I took a copy of the newspaper article with me. I discussed again with Lorna what had happened to her mood during chemo. She said she always got very tearful during the second weekend. This could have been due to withdrawal from dexamethasone.

Lorna's consultant came to see one of our patients. She was thrilled to see Lorna back at work and looking so well. We reintroduced ourselves to each other and I explained I was on docetaxol for breast cancer. I was tempted to ask her immediately about whether she had heard about the inquest into Jay Milne's death, but thought it would be tactless and inappropriate; however, she mentioned the use of dexamethasone, so I asked her if she had seen the article. She said she had. We agreed side-effects are often only discussed if the patient mentions the problem. I encouraged her to discuss it with her colleagues, pointing out Jay's father had been on the radio. I was really pleased we had had the conversation and she was also very encouraged. It was so helpful to discuss the issue. It was obviously on her mind, especially as so many of her patients have no choice but to take dexamethasone if they are to have life-prolonging chemotherapy.

I attended day hospice again in the afternoon as we were visited by Sue of Birds of Bray plus Whisper the barn owl and Moss the tawny owl. It was great to take photos of the patients again.

Friday 16 February
Reflection on mood swings

I chatted to Rachel (practice manager) at the surgery today. We talked about my mood swings. I told her that I know that my mood will become high again next Tuesday when I start back on dexamethasone and then it will drop again around about a week later, and so on. At least it's a regular cycle and eventually it will settle again. I realise how much worse it must be for those who suffer from bipolar affective disorder as they never know when the next mood swing is going to come along. No wonder they have such a high suicide rate. It is interesting to think that I consider I feel more inspired (because I am more reflective) when my mood is low rather than high, whereas people with bipolar disorder often thrive on the highs (provided they don't get out of control) because they get so much done and are more creative.

I am aware I am a little irritable today – more irritable than usual about Nick leaving his shoes in the middle of the lounge floor, for example.

I am also really troubled by hot flushes during the night and day. My sleep is really disturbed. At least I don't have to worry that I might be up all night working the following night.

Monday 19 February

I am struggling this evening. My veins aren't that good now. They failed to get enough blood from me today and now my left arm hurts! I hope they manage it tomorrow in the chemo unit. I wish I could take it myself. It reminded me of the time when Marian was a toddler and needed a drip because of her asthma. She was screaming and the SHO failed to insert the cannula even though she had excellent veins. I wished I had been able to do it myself.

I weighed myself at the weekend. This was an awful shock. I have suddenly put on nearly a stone. I am beginning to hate dexamethasone; it is causing so many problems, yet I have to take it again tomorrow. I have no choice.

I've cut out all sweets and biscuits and other snacks to try to control my weight and at least I managed to go on a couple of walks over the weekend. I'm really pleased with my photos of a male and a female goldeneye on Wilstone reservoir.

I walked along the canal at Broughton yesterday. It was a grey afternoon so it appeared to get dark earlier than expected. Even so, I had a wonderful view of a kingfisher for a good length of time. In fact, I watched the kingfisher on one side of the canal and a great spotted woodpecker in a tree on the other at the same time. I also saw several fieldfares flying over. As it got dark a sparrow hawk flew low over the canal and, as I walked back along the tow path, I looked at a dead tree trunk with holes in it, wondering what might be using it. As I watched a tawny owl flew out of a hole and landed in a near by tree. It was lovely to watch.

Just because it was a grey day, and today has been just the same, doesn't mean it is all dreary; there are moments of beauty and joy. It was good to walk beside the canal again and to pray and reflect. I knew when I started out on my journey back to health it was going to be a long one. I'm now halfway through my chemotherapy and it is beginning to feel like quite an ordeal. Having to face another three cycles of treatment is definitely not easy, and I know it will get harder. At least I have Easter and Spring Harvest to look forward to, after my last dose.

Tuesday 20 February

One of the nurses from the chemo unit managed to get my blood for the blood test but it was painful. I will go there from now on and let them use the bigger veins first!

I spent time in day hospice showing everyone the owl photos. It was so lovely to see the face of one of the older ladies light up with happiness, when she saw her picture.

I went to see Amanda in outpatients. My blood count is fine so I will have chemo tomorrow. I said I felt I really wasn't having problems with the chemo – just the dexamethasone. I briefly discussed the inquest report on the lad with the brain tumour but she hadn't seen it, so obviously hadn't thought out any of the implications – she understood why I had been distressed by it.

I started back on dexamethasone today. I really didn't want to but at least my weight this morning was under eleven stone. I must continue to cut out sugary snacks between meals. At least Lent starts tomorrow.

Wednesday – Ash Wednesday

I am so pleased that I managed to go to midweek communion today before going to chemo, especially as it is the beginning of Lent. I will try to go each week during Lent.

My last three doses of chemo are all in Lent. Lent isn't meant to be easy. We remember how Jesus fasted in the desert for forty days. Not an easy time, but a very special time, for him. I know the last three chemo cycles won't be easy, especially as I am also trying to watch my weight and I have been struggling with my mood, but at least I have Easter and Spring Harvest to look forward to at the end. I hope Spring Harvest can be a time of celebration and thanksgiving but also a time for reflection. We regularly go to Spring Harvest, the Easter Christian conference and holiday at Butlins, but this will be the first time I have been to Butlins with a disability.

I managed to get to the chemo unit on time and sat next to my friend having herceptin again. She had wondered where I was, so I explained that I had been to communion first.

It was good to compare notes. She also suddenly found she had put on a stone in weight in three weeks without noticing it. It is so easy to do with the drugs we have to take. She said she only became aware of her problem when she couldn't get her socks on – just like me! She was also breathless going upstairs, etc.

Phyllis was volunteering again. It was lovely to see her. She said she had been to a stately home to look round and the gardener was trimming the yew trees. He said all the branches would be used for the manufacture of cancer drugs. I was amused to think that my docetaxol – made from yew tree pine needles – might even be locally grown yew trees!

I even managed to get to our church home group meeting in the evening, which was lovely.

Thursday 22 February

This was a much quieter day. I didn't go out at all and slept most of the afternoon. I did manage to spend some time doing my theology course, which was rewarding.

Friday 23 February

I am beginning to realise how much harder it's getting. I woke up quite late this morning, and had a late bath. I couldn't decide what to do. Should I go for a walk, or to Tesco, or to the surgery? I eventually decided to go to the market and get fruit and vegetables. We needed to stock up, but I only realised how weak I was when I tried to carry the groceries back to the car. I needed at least six pauses, and my arms ached afterwards. Again, I slept most of the afternoon and really struggled to get out of bed once I woke up.

I sat and read the *Bucks Herald* for ages, eventually mustered up sufficient energy to do a bit of washing up, and prepare vegetables for tea, but came back up to bed just after 8 p.m. I only had about three hours today with any energy at all.

I know it will get better but I certainly feel poisoned at the moment!

Sunday 25 February

Well, I was more awake yesterday. I woke up feeling better having slept the best part of the previous fifty-six hours! I really am quite shocked at how weak I am getting. After all, on the Friday after my second dose of docetaxol, I went into the surgery and worked. I cleaned the kitchen floor once too! This time I staggered to and from the market, which was a mistake, and spent most of the rest of the time in bed. Thanks to the generous donation of ham for tea, cooked by Shirley, we ate something!

Spiritual reflection: God's laws and man-made rules

Whilst doing some tidying up this morning I found a computer print out of psalm 19 - an easy to read version. This helped to focus my mind, so I thought I would try to memorise part to help my reflection during the day. I love psalm 19.

The Heavens are telling the glory of God,
And the firmament (or skies above) proclaims his handiwork.

How true that is. As I walk or drive around day or night I am reminded of God's greatness and his amazing creativity. Each cloud formation is different, transient and so beautiful. I'll never forget the evening I was driving back from the surgery at Whitchurch towards Aylesbury and the sun was beginning to set. A beautiful cumulus cloud was illuminated perfectly by the pink setting sun. For a few moments I was amazed by its magnificence but then, as I drove on, the view disappeared. I praised the Lord for that moment of beauty and felt Him say, 'I did that for you.' What wonderful love. Yes, I was driving quickly and I was the only car on that stretch of road. Maybe I really was the only person who saw that and appreciated its transient, but amazing beauty. Every day there is something new to be marvelled at, a new creation.

I love the way psalm 19 moves from praise about God's mighty creation to reflection on His perfect law.

The Law of the Lord is perfect, reviving the soul.
The testimony of the Lord is sure, making wise the simple.

Yes, making wise the simple! If we read and meditate on His law (and the psalmist only had the first few books of the Old Testament) we grow in wisdom without having to be anything like intellectual giants. I've seen it happen so many times as well.

What a contrast between God's everlasting laws and man's tradition. Jesus challenged the rules of the Pharisees and scribes – their handwashing rituals, and strict regulations about what could and could not be done on the Sabbath, which excluded doing good.

I went into Aylesbury town yesterday to get a few jobs done. My glasses needed straightening – I was really struggling to read. They've been getting caught up in my hats and have become misshapen. It was lunchtime and I couldn't keep going without a rest.

Nick had gone off to support his team, Plymouth Argyle, playing at QPR, so I bought a pasty and sat in Friar's Square to eat it.

My mind wandered. I started to think about the difference between God's laws laid down thousands of years ago — and still true today — and a rule I had been given in our final term at medical school in 1979. I think this was probably the closest we ever got to being taught any medical ethics at medical school. Unfortunately, it wasn't about how we should treat others, our patients or our colleagues, but about how we should behave. We were going to be doctors, our patients would look up to us, set us on a pedestal, and we were to set an example. Dress code was very strict — that had to be modified for health and safety reasons as much as anything! The rule I remember most clearly causing great dismay among my peers was that we should never be seen eating fish and chips (or the equivalent) in the street, in case we bumped into a patient and set a bad example. We were going to be pillars of the community, and we needed to behave appropriately.

As I sat and ate my pasty in public, I wondered how many thousands of times I had broken that man-made rule! Life has changed so much since those days, but I still feel a little guilty if I'm in my local community and eating in the street. At least I would have had time to talk if someone had sat down next to me; I would not have rushed off in a hurry but had time to listen. Surely that is a better example for me to set, giving people time.

The male professor never mentioned how a young female doctor, but also a young mother, should behave. I breastfed discreetly in public. I am sure this was a good example. Also, should I have deprived my children of snacks whilst we were out because they were the children of a doctor and I should set a good example? I think the screams of frustration would have been much more unacceptable! This man-made rule is really just amusing now, twenty-eight years later but God's rules last forever.

This may just seem amusing but it is a worrying reflection on the attitude to the status of doctors in the past. I certainly looked at medicine as a vocation, a calling to serve and to help others. Were we taught to serve? Some of the hospital doctors showed wonderful caring qualities, whereas others expected the nurses and juniors to run around after them, obey their orders and never to have their demands challenged – or that was the image they projected.

Perhaps I am being very hard on my own medical school; I loved it and flourished there in so many ways, but we know that not every doctor learnt to serve acceptably.

Unfortunately there are plenty of examples of doctors, in this country from a variety of different medical schools and backgrounds, who have practised unacceptably. Of course, Harold Shipman was the most appalling example of a single-handed practitioner who only gave his doting patients the impression that he was serving them. His patients set him on a pedestal and he murdered them. Of course there are wonderful examples of single-handed practitioners who are great GPs, but it is so much easier to cover up bad practice when you are not working with others.

In my own experience, if only my former partner, who had previously worked on his own, had learnt to work as a member of a team, to respect the opinion of others, to treat others as he would have them treat himself, rather than expecting them to do exactly what he said. The belief that he was the boss, and patients and staff looked up to him, ultimately seemed to me to mean that, in his eyes, it was all right for patients to think of him as 'god', and for him to 'lord it' over those who worked for him. All his arrogant, behaviour was acceptable in his eyes; he could behave like a bully and get away with it. This is what I felt he was expressing as he shouted at me on my leaving day, as we were in his consulting room, with the door closed, and he was moving threateningly towards me: 'This is my surgery, my building, my staff, my patients and my room, and in my room I can do whatever I like.'

We need to serve; all he used to do was insist on being served. It was very easy for a small practice, with one overbearing authoritarian doctor in control, to conceal misdemeanours. His wife, as practice manager, rarely employed anyone as a member of the clerical or reception staff who had worked in a similar job, so they always had to be trained and supervised by her, and had no preconceived ideas about what is normal or acceptable within general practice.

In Mark 10: 42–45 Jesus talks about the rulers of the gentiles lording it over the people, and exercising authority over them, as an example of unacceptable 'greatness'. Instead, he said to his disciples that to become great we must learn to serve. Jesus set us that example to follow today.

March 2007

Wednesday 1 March – St David's Day

This has been a very hard week; I have been so weak and tired I haven't had the time or the energy to sit down and write my journal.

I found Tuesday particularly exhausting. It was hard working at the hospice in the morning. I couldn't believe how exhausting it was to walk from the doctor's office to day hospice. It showed me how good a patient is if they can walk to the front door! I wanted to have time to do some mosaic work but I struggled to get to day hospice before lunch. It would have been very unsociable not to sit with the patients at lunchtime but then it's their rest time. I eventually managed to sit down at the craft table at 2.20 p.m.

All I wanted to do was sleep when I got home but I did manage to do some studying in the evening.

I tried to have a restful day today, aware I was covering the police for Aylesbury but I kept feeling guilty that I wasn't at the surgery doing paperwork, even though I would have struggled to concentrate. I was eventually called to the police station at 4 p.m. Although I had been feeling very tired it was good to go to the police station. The custody sergeant wanted to have a chat and Angie, now a drugs rehabilitation worker, was there. I hadn't seen her for months and hadn't realised she was no longer a jailer. It was good to spend time there. I was encouraged; I helped a prisoner, and gained from the company. I eventually stopped feeling guilty about not going to the surgery; after all I was on call for the police.

Friday 2 March

I had a chat with another doctor today who went through chemo and radiotherapy two years ago, and who reduced her workload greatly as a result. As she said to me: 'If you do get to eighty you won't look back and think "if only I had done an extra night on call when I was working".' But of course we might well regret being too busy post-diagnosis to make the most of the time when we are well. It was nice to hear someone else talking very practically about making sure her husband knows how to do the housework!

I spent time doing theology course work and watched two DVDs today. *Tsotsi* was an incredibly powerful movie filmed in Soweto; I am so glad I made time to watch it.

Saturday 3 March

I slept badly again, with a lot of hot flushes, but the sun was shining all day and it was a beautifully clear night. The perfect night for a total eclipse of the moon!

I went for a walk in the early afternoon. Wilstone was incredibly muddy and it tried to rain for a short time. There was a wonderful rainbow arching over the reservoir. Highlights were five snipe in the reeds by the hide and I definitely saw a firecrest in the trees around the hide. It was preening so I could see its fiery head and stripe through its eye very clearly. I also heard my first chiffchaff of the year.

I went up to London with Nick and our friend Brigette to have a meal and then see the play Marian was in: *The Tolstoy Tales*. We thoroughly enjoyed the production with some extremely funny moments and some very profound. I am looking forward to seeing it again on Friday with Rachel.

Rachel is having a difficult weekend – overwhelmed by all the things she has to do. I wish I could help her more. She's so far away when she is distressed; talking over the phone doesn't seem to be enough.

Sunday 4 March

After the performance last night we went to the pub with Marian and then looked at the 'blood-red moon'. I took some photos of it as the shadow began to move away after midnight when we got home. On three occasions in twenty-four hours I regretted not having my camera with me!

I gave Elaine a big hug in church today during the service. I am so glad I saw her – she is struggling post-lumpectomy. She asked me if it is OK to be weepy. I said of course it was! Sometimes it isn't helpful if I come over as always being cheerful. She felt guilty that she wasn't. I will ring her again this week.

Tuesday 6 March

I had a busy but successful day yesterday – on call for the police for Aylesbury and doing paperwork at the surgery.

I had a better day today at the hospice with a lovely time in day hospice in the afternoon doing my mosaic.

Spiritual reflection

I am really enthused by my theology course now. Reflecting on the last seven recorded sentences of Jesus on the cross has been really inspiring. He showed his compassion by praying for his persecutors, talking tenderly to his mother and beloved apostle John, and to the penitent thief. Apart from the ultimate triumphant cry 'IT IS FINISHED', the other three 'words' from the cross are quotations from the psalms. It is a beautiful thought that for me the psalms are my greatest comfort when I am really stressed, and the really human Jesus, suffering agony on the cross, was also obtaining consolation from the psalms.

My God, my God, why hast thou forsaken me?

Is the first verse of psalm 22. In verses 6 to 8 the psalmist talks of being despised, mocked, and insults hurled at him. It is hard to read verse 8 without singing, using the words of the oratorio The Messiah:

He trusted in God, let him deliver him, for he delights in him.

Verses 16 to 17 describe so completely what was happening to Jesus:

They have pierced my hands and feet – I can count all my bones;

On the cross his whole body would have hurt and it would have become more and more difficult to breathe.

Jesus hanging from the cross was watching as

They divide my garments among them and for my raiment they cast lots (verse 18).

What about those around the cross, watching him die? They heard Jesus quoting the psalm. The Jews, whether they loved him or hated him, would have known the psalm. Those who loved him would see the clear link between the suffering of Jesus and the psalmist's prophecy. Those who had condemned him might have been challenged by the description of themselves, or it might have just made them more antagonistic.

Thursday 8 March

I had a successful time at the hospice. I definitely heard two skylarks singing in the field.

I travelled to London after lunch. I got to Marylebone carrying gifts for my mother's birthday, but was determined to walk to Regent's Park. I spotted a magnolia in full bloom on the way – surely this is very early? I was breathless with a very fast pulse by the time I reached the park, but it was worth it. The gardens were full of daffodils, tulips, primroses and other flowers. I saw plenty of herons on nests and pochard, red-crested pochard, great-crested grebe and a merganser on the lake plus several coots on nests.

I wanted to go to Piccadilly to buy some fruit tea before going to Victoria. I made the mistake of changing trains at Green Park – there were several short flights of stairs rather than an escalator. This was hard work, especially with very swollen ankles.

I had a good time with mum and my brother-in-law Chris, celebrating her seventy-sixth birthday. She is moving pretty well post-left knee replacement after Christmas. She is much fitter than me at present!

Friday 9 March

I met Rachel at Euston station at 6.30 p.m. We enjoyed an excellent Indian meal before seeing Marian's play again. I am so pleased so many of her friends, and several of our church, went to see it and enjoyed it. Rachel seems more relaxed this week.

Sunday 11 March

I walked to church this morning. It was so warm and sunny and all the gardens were looking so colourful. One lawn was covered in violets. I certainly wasn't expecting that!

The weather was so good that I went to Wilstone reservoir in the afternoon. It was much less muddy than last week. I managed to photograph four snipe close to the hide. They were still in the same place as last week! The walk to and from the hide was far enough today even though it really isn't very far!

Oh dear – Plymouth Argyle lost in the quarter-finals of the FA cup this evening, but at least Nick was at the match.

Monday 12 March

Today is my sister Christine's birthday. It will be great to celebrate it with her this evening. She's flown over from California.

I spent two hours in surgery today doing telephone consultations. It has been so good just talking to patients again. It has been very therapeutic and, of course, I have been able to go at my own pace. Patients have wanted to chat and find out how I am getting on, and I have had some good discussions with other ladies with breast cancer; one in particular had only had a mastectomy three weeks ago. I did not know she had breast cancer. It was really constructive talking about prostheses and chemotherapy, etc.

Tuesday 13 March

It was great to see my sister Christine and her husband Chris last night. We picked a little village pub from the *Good Beer Guide*, just off the M11 somewhere between Suffolk and Aylesbury, but had little idea whether the food would be good enough. It turned out to be just right and we had a good chat. I hadn't realised she had been thinking about having a breast enhancement operation – at least she was looking at prices and researching it – in Thailand, when I told her I had breast cancer. She decided it would be inappropriate in the circumstances, and certainly insensitive. I don't think I would have been offended, but I'm not sure it would have been wise – we'll see.

Reflection on being a patient

I had to be honest today; it would have been foolish not to be.

I was very breathless, and my pulse rate 120, when I walked from the hospice to the chemo unit at lunchtime, and I had been noticeably breathless just walking from the new car park first thing. Colleagues said I looked exhausted and I had only just arrived.

I am really not looking forward to another round of chemo, and all the side-effects, but I only have to look at Lorna, and how well and active she is now, to think I am being a coward. Maybe I'm being a bit harsh on myself as this is my fifth cycle of docetaxol, but my seventh chemo cycle, and my body is saying it's had enough!

I had my oncology outpatient appointment today, and Amanda asked me if I was beginning to feel I didn't really want any more. I said, 'Yes, but I would have the next lot, but then review the situation.' Most of the benefit is gained from the first four treatments so it wouldn't be too bad to only have five. I expect I will go through with all six, however, as I don't want to let my family down. Helen, my palliative care consultant, thinks I will, as I am too stubborn to give in!

I didn't compose a list of questions for Amanda prior to my appointment, but did scribble down three things just before she called me in. I often find it irritating when patients come in with a long list of questions when I know it's a ten-minute appointment. I did remember to talk about the most troublesome symptom – breathlessness – and we agreed that I should try a diuretic (water tablet). I also remembered to ask about the timing of radiotherapy in relation to our planned June holiday. I think we will manage to fit it in, with a few days to spare, but I will be sore. If nothing else I will be able to sit and watch the estuary, and enjoy some short walks and good food!

By not writing a list I forgot to mention the allergic reaction that developed at the site of the cannula. Never mind, we will see what happens tomorrow – the dexamethasone will prevent any major reaction.

Typically, although I had put them in an obvious place this morning, I forgot to take my first dose of dexamethasone before going to work this morning. Fortunately, I remembered on the way so could obtain some when I got there. I wonder how many people forget but aren't in the same position as me, having access to a dispensary at work. It is much more difficult to remember to commence a treatment the day before chemo, than to continue it afterwards!

Wednesday 14 March

It's chemotherapy day today – Docetaxol cycle number five.

Yesterday I was dreading it – I was so breathless and knew it was only going to get worse. Today I am more positive; I know I will be able to walk further; I am definitely less oedematous (swollen).

Following 20 mg furosemide, I have just been up and downstairs three times quite quickly, with little distress. This is better! I did pass urine in larger volumes yesterday afternoon, and overnight, but not excessively. In fact I lost 2 kg over the last twenty-four hours – that's two litres of fluid, a very significant amount! Of course, starting back on dexamethasone will have reduced its effect, but at least there was a better balance. By yesterday evening my left arm was significantly more comfortable, and my veins visible. This should be an advantage for the nurses this morning!

Nick noticed the telangectasia (tiny blood vessels) on my cheeks have become obvious again overnight – one day of dexamethasone and I have red cheeks again. I trust they will settle again quickly.

My mood seems better today. I'm not high, but suddenly rather more creative again, and wanting to write up my journal. I lay in bed for a while during the night thinking of new ideas, and thoughts to reflect on, for this journal, and for my write-up of the saga of my former practice. Unfortunately, the journal has also taken second place, as I have been trying to keep up with my theology module coursework. I have so many things to reflect on now, it is so rewarding, but I need time to get it down in writing. The course has the advantage of set deadlines. I am so much better working to deadlines!

This journal now has its first deadline. My radiotherapy is due to start on 30 April and finish at the beginning of June. Perhaps that is when I should try to finish it.

Ethical reflection on palliative care

I woke up this morning thinking about two conversations I have had at the hospice during my last two sessions there.

The more I think about it, the more amused and amazed I am about how relevant my ethics dissertation was to my present life as a doctor, but also a patient. I concluded my dissertation emphasising the importance of carefully listening to the hospice patient and making it clear that I had time to listen, I'm not in a hurry, and I'm not planning to run away. In order to do this I resolved to sit down by the bedside – something that needs to be taught to the juniors – positioning the chair to maintain good eye contact, on the patient's good side, for example.

As my chemotherapy has progressed and I have become weaker, the patients and relatives are more often noticing my illness, and sitting down has become an essential, anyway. My puffy face and variety of hats are a bit of a give away too!

One patient with increasing abdominal swelling due to bowel obstruction had been deteriorating over a week or so. I went to have a chat with her with the senior house officer (junior doctor) last Thursday. The SHO pointed out that the one thing that hadn't been tried was a short course of dexamethasone, but she had refused this when offered, although it might give some hope. The patient was only a little older than me so I sat down with her, with my swollen ankles and puffy face, and brought up the subject again. It was good to have the SHO there, as she felt it was constructive teaching (and she always makes sure I have a chair).

I asked the patient about her fears. She said she was concerned about having a puffy face again. When she had had chemo before, and was on dexamethasone, she hadn't liked it. I acknowledged the fact that I too dislike having a puffy face, but what is more important? An hour or so later, with the support of her family she agreed to try a course of dexamethasone to see if it would help resolve her bowel obstruction. I made it very clear to them all that this provided hope, but I could make no promises of success.

From an ethical point of view I was happy I had obtained informed consent. I demonstrated guided autonomy to the SHO by acknowledging the patient's fears and I know this made a difference. I was being the doctor but with the experience of being a patient, and the message was clear. It was important for her not to give up hope, but it was also important to gently question the reasoning behind her previous apparently autonomous decisions not to have the treatment. The unspoken message behind the gentle questioning was really: 'Is it better to have a puffy face or die without one last fight?'

Yesterday (five days later), I chatted to her again to see how we were getting on. Had there been any improvement? She had been getting severe labour-type colicky abdominal pains and nausea. She said that these had settled over the last few days and she was much more comfortable. The dexamethasone had helped to make her much more comfortable. However much I dislike taking the drug, it can be extremely helpful. This was good palliative care.

The other patient who made me think was a man who had a tumour removed, and for some years was disease-free. He believed he was cured and then suddenly developed a recurrence. This was a real blow for him.

He is finding it very hard to adjust, as he wasn't expecting to die yet. This made me think about my cancer. It is important to plan for the future but also learn to live with the uncertainty. As long as the Lord wants me here on earth, my daughters and husband need me, and I can serve my patients, I want to be here, but please don't let me become useless. Dying of breast cancer sometime in the future may not be pleasant, but at least I would know what is going on and have some insight.

My chemo went very well today, and I even went to communion and popped into the hospice afterwards, to prove how much further I could walk. I think I will have a quiet evening, though!

Thursday 15 March

I made the right decision not to go out yesterday evening. I had a significant amount of oesophageal (chest) pain, and certainly would have had to come home. It was good just to relax and watch *MasterChef* on television. It's the final tonight, so I will do the same again.

I had a leisurely morning, but managed to get to my theology tutorial after looking through my notes for the four topics. There were only two of us today, plus Mike our tutor, so my decision to try not to talk too much, but let others do the talking, didn't work this time; of course it didn't matter. It was good to talk about the psalms Jesus quoted from the cross, and to reflect that during times of suffering, the psalms are all I feel I am able to read. Mike mentioned others who had had the same experience, and reminded me that the 'blackest' of psalms – with no feeling of hope – is psalm 88, but it helps to remind us that things could be worse!

Later in the tutorial I talked a bit about my time of endurance at the dysfunctional practice, and then Mike told one of his funny stories. I was amazed and must mention it to him next time, as he has no idea what it meant to me!

He said that it was Nero's birthday, and he decided to have a party to celebrate. He chose a few Christians to crucify. Whilst they were suffering in front of him on the cross, he asked one if he wanted to say anything. He replied 'Happy birthday!' We laughed, but Mike said it did reveal great love (compassion) on the part of the sufferer. I was speechless (very unusual) thinking, 'but that's what I did on that last day I worked at that practice'. It was meant to be my penultimate, day but became my last day after I wished the practice manager 'happy birthday' and she went out of control as a result, throwing the post everywhere and hurling abuse at me. She was the one who was really frightened, though as she must have realised she was out of control, and summoned her husband in to sort me out when she realised I was serious about involving the police. My lasting memory of her – the last time I saw her at that surgery – was of her running upstairs, following her husband, hunched, tiny, terrified, fleeing. What I saw was not the manager of the practice but the wicked witch (queen), as painted by Disney, in *Snow White*, fleeing from the scene as the princess revives – or, at least, my memory of the film!

When I wished her 'happy birthday' it triggered all that; it was impossible for her to accept that I could be polite or nice to her. She certainly could not reciprocate. (See 'Play within the play' for further details)

Friday 16 March

Red nose day!

I enjoyed a restful evening watching the *MasterChef* final, and Ireland tying their first-ever world cup cricket match. It was great fun to watch, except that they were playing Zimbabwe. After the appalling beating of the leader of the opposition, and many others arrested at a prayer meeting on Sunday and outside the police station later in the day, it is very hard to know what to think watching the Zimbabwean team. I can read about the suffering, and pray for regime change, but should they even be allowed to have a team playing, in the circumstances? What do the players themselves think? It must be an awful time for them, with the economy failing, and hearing this sort of news, where it can be talked about much more freely.

When I woke up this morning it was before 7 a.m., so I had my medication and dozed back to sleep, thinking that I would have a cup of coffee if someone brought me one! I did in fact make one, and then went back to bed. Nick woke me as he shouted 'goodbye' on his way to work at about 8.40 a.m. I got up and made myself breakfast and found the paper. I thought I ought to have a shower, but I took my breakfast and the paper back to bed, already feeling quite exhausted. I tried to read the paper, but struggled to concentrate, so I lay down again to see what would happen. I remember thinking that if I were in the hospice, and one of the nurses told me a bath had been run for me, and all I had to do was get out of bed, and into a wheelchair, I would have got up! That, of course didn't happen, and the next thing I was aware of was hearing the cuckoo clock. I wondered if it was 10, or maybe 11 a.m. already, but in fact it was

12, I had slept for another three hours. I realised I was feeling a lot more energetic.

I showered and rang my mother. I felt alert and well enough, to drive to the hospice for a special 'red lunch' organised by Dorothy, one of the nurses. As I drove there, I was dreaming of the promised summer pudding. It definitely lived up to expectations. I must start making them, especially as this one was made by Dorothy's husband and was perfect.

I joked at two o'clock that it was time for me to have another nap, and came home. This definitely needs to be a very quiet day, but I realised that I could watch the cricket for a while – England v New Zealand – so rested in front of the television instead!

Medication and symptom review

I resolved that I would rest again at 4 p.m., but failed to drop off to sleep, turned over onto my left side, and realised I had pain in my left hip and couldn't lie on that side. Time for a medication review – what have I taken today; have I forgotten anything?

When I woke early I took 30 mg lansoprazole. This I need to manage the oesophageal pain (mucositis) and to protect my stomach lining from ulceration, which can occur with dexamethasone and ibuprofen. I also took 10 mg metoclopramide as an anti-emetic. I wasn't feeling sick, but better to take it before developing nausea, than struggle to keep an anti-sickness drug down!

Of course I took my inhalers – salbutamol and Serevent and my nasal spray Flixonase. These are routine for my asthma and allergic rhinitis, and nothing to do with my cancer treatment.

I remembered to take 4 mg dexamethasone when I got up again at twelve o'clock. Today, 4 mg and 2 mg tomorrow and Sunday to tail off the drug slowly, to try to avoid the huge dip in mood I had after my second dose of docetaxol. I didn't notice a real dip during the last cycle, but I was so weak, and then so swollen, that I wasn't really aware of my mood until I felt 'normal' again on Tuesday, after I had restarted the dexamethasone. I wonder what will happen this time – maybe it will be more affected by the cricket than the drugs!

I know my muscles are weak, and this morning I tried to open my bowels, but realised that it would be impossible to strain at all. I would need to be patient, or at least take some more laxative, as I could soon become constipated again, and I don't want another awful weekend. Therefore, I had another sachet of Movicol this afternoon. I hope I don't get too much colic overnight. I took a sachet on Wednesday and one yesterday. That was enough last cycle, but of course I'm weaker this time, and it will be the same next time. Good news, though – I have managed to open my bowels a little this afternoon!

When I developed hip pain I took 400 mg ibuprofen. I will need to take more at bed-time to treat the joint pains I will get, and the pain in my fingers and toes due to the transient peripheral neuropathic type pain I get each cycle. Fortunately, I seem to be able to control it with ibuprofen, and it resolves before the next dose.

The other thing I have noticed is a strange smell, which may be an odour due to me getting rid of the docetaxol. What do metabolised yew tree pine needles smell like? I have decided to take some fluconazole and have a short course of anti-thrush treatment in case that's the real cause.

This evening I will take another metoclopramide, and probably just take it if necessary tomorrow. I will have another lansoprazole

30 mg but hopefully I won't need any antacids overnight. I will take more ibuprofen at bedtime, and my inhalers and a sleeping tablet to enable me to get sleep. That sounds absurd as I have been so sleepy today, but the dexamethasone keeps my mind active, and I don't want to be composing my journal all night!

What a list! No wonder patients get confused. At least I can cut down the drugs over the next few days, and have permission to do so. I am not self-medicating, but I am allowed to be in control. I am so privileged to understand what does what, and what can cause the side-effects I have.

I weighed myself this morning. I have lost nearly 3 kg since taking 20 mg furosemide on Tuesday afternoon. What a difference that has made! I'm nothing like as breathless and I'm not aware of my heart racing as I walk upstairs. My ankles are comfortable and not puffy, my arms and hands are no longer swollen, and my skirt is loose. Three litres of fluid is quite a significant amount, and it is heavy!

What's causing the pain in my left thigh? Why has it come on? It seems to be the outer aspect of the femur rather than the hip itself. Is it the chemo working? What does that mean? Does it mean I do have bony spread? I have tried not to think like that but I am a doctor, and I knew I would think like that sometimes. I always get aches and pains when the dexamethasone is reduced. I am sure that is the real cause, and my ribs are a bit uncomfortable as well. It is far more likely to be a transient joint pain, and nothing to worry about.

Reflection on my past work problems – my time at a very dysfunctional practice

I have spent years trying to work out the best way to tell my story concisely. Where should I begin the story so it's not too boring? Writing it up like a diary could be very tedious. I wanted to write a summary or short testimony, to set the scene so that later reflections could be put in context. This week the solution came to me: I realised it would flow well if I started at the moment when I resigned, and then explain why and what happened subsequently. I wanted to produce a concise account, not just for my reflective write-up, which may or may not ever be published, but also as a simple but coherent statement for use on my theology course, and within my church.

Is it reasonable to identify the name of the practice? No, I shouldn't, I must change the names, but the practice has changed beyond recognition anyway. In fact it is wonderful to think that after all my traumas a new practice now serves and meets those patients' needs. It makes me feel that what I went through was really worthwhile.

What I am writing at present is my experience and my interpretation of what happened to me, and I am giving my opinion as to the causes. I will call the doctor and his wife Dr and Mrs C to disguise their surname which really begins with another letter of the alphabet.

I am aware I have reflected on my time at the surgery over the last few months in this journal, but I will include the concise summary at this point, as I finally wrote it this week, followed by further in-depth reflections. In addition, this is the appropriate place to insert my other reflections. It's the story within my story but as so much has been written up in the style of a drama. I will call it the 'play within the play'.

The play within the play – the dysfunctional practice

Introduction

At the beginning of March, when my daughters were at middle school, I resigned from my partnership in general practice. It was a small practice with just two doctors. I had been working there for seventeen months. I did not resign because we were moving, or I had a better job to go to, but solely because I could no longer work with the practice manager. I was very unhappy about the way she treated our staff, and her behaviour was unacceptable. Unfortunately, I had no control over her, although as her employer I was responsible for her actions, and I could not discipline her or ask her to leave as she was the wife of my GP partner, who always supported her. I had no choice but to leave myself.

One example of her unacceptable behaviour occurred three months after I joined the practice. I discovered that a letter had been written by my GP partner's wife, in the name of the practice, to a volunteer who helped us once a week to inform her that she had been replaced. This was the first the volunteer knew about it.

I knew nothing about it until I heard that she had been so upset it had made her very ill. On asking my partner for an explanation, I was told I had not been working there long enough to question what went on. I never saw a copy of the letter, and I was told his wife wrote 'good letters'. Since it made the volunteer ill, I had serious doubts about this.

When I resigned I was meant to work six months' notice. With legal advice I managed to reduce this to three months. It would have been impossible to work there any longer. The manager's behaviour did not improve; in fact it grew worse and worse. On a positive note, at least whilst I was there she mostly directed her rage at me, so I deflected her appalling behaviour away from my staff. For weeks after I left, although I was greatly relieved, I felt very guilty that I was no longer there to protect the rest of the team, and I knew she would be attacking someone else.

By the time I left I had been shouted at, sworn at repeatedly and my faith mocked. The manager used to wait outside my consulting room and burst into the room between patients to hurl abuse at me. I then had to see and concentrate on the next patient, trying to forget about what had just been said. On one occasion when I said 'good morning' to her in the reception area, in front of patients, receptionists and her husband, she just spat. Her husband stood there watching and said nothing. One day she drove rapidly into the car park and straight into a parking space without waiting, even though I was standing in it at the time, forcing me to move quickly out of the way. She would push past me in doorways and shut the door in my face.

Until I had experienced this type of treatment, I had no idea how lonely it is to be branded the enemy. I felt I was being terrorised but had no-one I could safely turn to for support. Although my colleagues, especially the nursing staff, secretly supported me as they observed what was going on, and had seen it all before, by the time it came to the last week they had to appear to be supporting the manager in everything she did, or risk losing their jobs.

The manager was desperate to provoke me into retaliating in some way, but because of my faith I had the excellent example of Jesus, the suffering servant, to follow. It worked! I accepted the abuse but never lifted a finger against either the manager or her husband; I never retaliated so they never had anything substantial against me. They did make up some charges. I was accused, with evidence, of being too honest, and when I left, I heard they informed patients who enquired that they had got rid of me because I was too religious, and kept preaching at them. Well, it is true that I made it clear when I believed what was going on was unethical, or even contrary to employment law, but it was important to make a stand.

One year after I left the practice, I received a letter from them that provided all the evidence I needed to confirm what I said had been happening, but that was just my word against theirs; this was written evidence.

The letter described me, among other things, as 'the nastiest, most vindictive and wicked person ever to walk this earth' and also 'dog shit' that needed to be removed from their shoes – 'unfortunately the smell remains'. It was clearly composed by the manager but it was signed by her husband, my former GP partner, and copied to the legal adviser at the British Medical Association. I was astonished at their lack of insight. The sort of letter they had written really said nothing about my character but completely exposed them.

This was the example of a 'good letter' I had been waiting for. I never saw the letter sent to the volunteer, but if this 'good letter' was anything to go by, no wonder she became ill. This sort of thing had been going on behind my back, but in the name of the partnership. I was definitely right to leave when I did. I have no idea how often letters like this were sent to people, but I have spoken to patients over the years since I left, who also received distressing correspondence and unacceptable telephone calls from my former partner and his wife.

My resignation

I had been a partner in the practice seventeen months when I finally concluded that I was no longer prepared to work with Mrs C as my practice manager. I was not criticising her computer and general administrative skills, but we were a small practice and she was unacceptable as a personnel manager. I was her boss and ultimately responsible (along with her husband) for her performance, decisions and behaviour, but I could not discuss or reason with her. She argued with me, shouted at me, and had stormed out of a meeting when I was disagreeing with her saying I was 'the most impossible person' she had ever worked with. In all my professional life I had never argued like this with anyone. In fact, the last time I had argued like that was when I was a child, squabbling with my sisters, and then one of us would run to our mother to sort it all out. In the surgery setting that was exactly what was happening; when she didn't get her way, she would run to her husband to sort me out. Her behaviour appeared so childish. When I tried to raise the issue with her, she seemed to think that this was normal, telling me that I hadn't been in a management position before.

My concern was not so much her behaviour towards me, but how she was destroying the self-esteem of those working with us. As a Christian I was not prepared to work with someone who deliberately chose not to 'treat others as you would have them treat you', or not to 'love your neighbour as yourself'. Alternatively, from a philosophical point of view, in Kantian terms, she failed to observe the practical imperative to treat people 'never simply as a means, but always at the same time as an end'; in other words to show respect for others. The staff was being 'used'; treated solely as a 'means' to a profit rather than special people. They were being devalued.

I explained to Dr C that I was happy to continue in partnership with him, but did not wish to work with his wife any more. This, as I knew it would be, was not an option. I tried to explain my reasons but he was not prepared to listen. I had no choice but to resign, but there was no compromise; he expected me to work my notice (officially for six months but finally only three) alongside the woman who, I had stated, I could not work with any longer.

I knew he hadn't listened, and felt he didn't care, as he then asked his wife to compose the letter to accept my resignation, as if I were one of his employees that he was happy to get rid of, rather than a professional partner. The fact that his wife wrote the letter deeply offended me, as it was because of her behaviour that I had resigned. Needless to say, there was nothing in the letter to say that I had achieved anything of value whilst working in the practice. In spite of my very real grievances Dr C was adamant that I had to honour the partnership agreement, and work six months' notice. I was warned discreetly by one of the nurses, who had witnessed the managers behaviour following the resignation of others, that her behaviour would 'get worse' towards me as I worked my notice, and the last few days would be particularly difficult.

Clearly Dr C had not told his wife the reason for my resignation. Her behaviour towards me did deteriorate further. Her room was on the second floor (in the roof) at the top of a very steep flight of stairs. Immediately after my resignation, at the end of a very difficult conversation, she screamed at me to get out of the room, and then chased me downstairs.

I was extremely frightened by this behaviour, I could have been seriously injured if I had tripped, but subsequently, on many occasions over the next three months, wondered if it might have been better if I had tripped. At least I would have been able to leave immediately, and I would have had clear evidence of her appalling behaviour, but my story might not have been believed.

After this incident I sought professional and legal help to enable me to leave the practice after three rather than six months, three months' notice being deemed sufficient by the local health authority.

Fortunately, my own general practitioner believed my story and could see how stressed I had become. He provided me with a medical certificate to sign me off work, citing 'stress' as the reason, if I wished to use it.

At this point I had a choice: should I work my notice or allow myself to have time off? What would the consequences be? What did I want to achieve?

I sought further advice and the words that stuck in my mind were, 'I don't think people should go off sick if they aren't', but the adviser also offered his expertise to try to help me; he repeatedly emphasised my need to stay 'whiter than white', however, so that my partner and his wife would have nothing significant to use against me.

I was deeply concerned that history would repeat itself when I left. Eye witnesses had discreetly advised me that the female partner I had replaced had been heard crying in her room as she struggled to cope with the level of stress.

If I went off sick, I could avoid further direct confrontation with Dr and Mrs C. This would reduce my level of stress, and my family's suffering, but was it an appropriate long-term solution?

If I left under those circumstances Dr and Mrs C could tell the patients and the health authority that I couldn't cope with the pressure of the work, and would be able to replace me without having to account for their actions.

I felt that the behaviour I was experiencing was so bad that I should try to prevent any other doctor being put through the same ordeal. As I had completely failed to change the attitude of either the doctor or his wife I chose to stay, enduring further insults, to try to reach a point where they would either concede that what was going on was wrong, or be held to account for their actions.

I had no idea what would happen, and I could not have worked the next three months without the support of professional colleagues, my family, church and many friends.

Did I make the right decision?

I survived but suffered a great deal mentally, emotionally and physically. Of equal concern was the effect it had on the rest of the staff who witnessed what was going on, but could say nothing if they wished to keep their own jobs. Some were incredibly supportive and phoned me in secret at home in the evening, but they were all frightened of what might happen to them.

What shocked and amazed me was the apparent level of fear expressed by the professionals outside the practice who were trying to help me. No-one doubted my story, but there was a distinct reluctance to get involved beyond advising me.

Although my husband was very supportive I was determined to avoid a confrontation between him and the doctor as they might have ended up fighting. I suspect this was the fear of the other professionals as well.

In spite of the trauma, I believe I made the right decision, but I never recommend that course of action to patients who come to see me in practice with a story of bullying in the workplace. I always assure them that I will sign them off work, for as long as they need. This is almost invariably until they have found another job and worked their notice. Their mental health improves dramatically as soon as they have had two to four weeks away from the pressure. I am very concerned by the number of people I see who experience bullying from management at work.

I always believe their stories, and seek to assure them that they had made the right decision to come and see me. The relief on their faces is a pleasure to see. Subsequently, it is enormously satisfying to see them start to flourish again as they rebuild their lives.

I believe 'whistle-blowing' in my situation was essential. Patient care was being jeopardised. A woman that is prepared to shout abuse at a doctor between consultations, when there is no time to recover their composure before seeing the next patient, is deliberately trying to provoke them into making a mistake. Under that level of stress – constantly worrying what would happen following the next consultation – how can anyone concentrate on the patient's problems? How can they discern any underlying psychological problems? The art of the consultation is in carefully listening and watching the patient, and having the wisdom to ask the right questions to carefully steer the consultation on the right course. How can you do that when you are preoccupied with something that has just occurred, and worried what will happen next? Will she barge in again between patients and throw something, or shout incoherently?

When I started at the practice I was surprised by the level of unmet and undetected psychological need within the patient population, and wondered why. Of course this was the situation; the previous female partner had probably been under a similar level of stress so, again, would not have been able to concentrate adequately during the consultation to discern the psychological needs of the patients. A practice that is failing to meet the needs of the patients has to change. A practice that is causing harm to the patients has to change rapidly.

I was told the manager's behaviour would deteriorate, and it did. On one occasion when I said 'good morning' to her in the reception area she replied by spitting. This took place in front of the receptionists and in clear view of the patients. Her husband stood by the door watching but said nothing. I was expected to start surgery pretending nothing had happened. But the pressure was at its worst the week before I left.

On the Friday before I left, just before morning surgery, she had been in and out of my room several times shouting abuse, mocking my religious belief, shouting at the top of her voice. I pointed out to her that there were patients in the waiting room and the door was open, but she was completely out of control.

Mrs C: We realise now how we have escaped a fate worse than death by you leaving!

We've only got anywhere by fighting, and now we've got rid of you!

Hazel: Please would you leave my room [the consulting room]?

Mrs C: No *'my* room'; no it's *my* room, you're only using it out of sufferance.

Mrs C [stamping her foot]: No, it's my room – you're still sulking because we didn't let you buy in [to purchase a share of the building, which she owned jointly with her husband].

Mrs C: You said you felt called to this place! Where's your God now? Is he talking to you? I'm strong because I rejected all that!

Hazel: Please would you leave the room?

As she left the room I thought, 'No, He's not talking to me but He is giving me a big hug!'

I was at my lowest point – at rock bottom, desperate for help and at that moment I was overwhelmed by a feeling of love – being loved by God. I was given the strength to carry on.

She left but returned throwing a screwed up ball of paper at me.

Mrs C: By the way, I thought you would like to know that our new partner is better qualified than you, and so much nicer.

(I specially noted the comment 'our' new partner as this summed up the situation, and the way she thought. It was not her husband's new partner it was 'our' partner. She had to be in control.)

Mrs C [continuing to rant]: You're so jealous and envious and you'll never get another job, when they know you walked out on your contract, you'll never get another job.

Hazel: I already have one.

Again, I asked her to leave. As she refused, but had slammed the door shut, I stood up to leave the room myself. She barred my way, dancing from side to side, like a goalkeeper defending a goal, and then using her fists like a boxer preparing a punch. She trapped me up against the hand basin. As I was determined to stay 'whiter than white' she was never going to entice me to fight her. I knew what would happen if I did raise my fist against her – she would run to her husband, and I had come to fear that greatly, even though I had no clear evidence of what might happen.

My room was in a recently built extension. Before I started using the room I pointed out to the practice manager that there was no emergency buzzer in the room. She had been involved in drawing up the plans for the room, and had chosen to omit this safety feature. On that Friday I discovered why. If I had had a buzzer I could have raised the alarm, and she would not have had the opportunity to treat me like that. Fortunately, the practice nurse knocked on the door and opened it as Mrs C had me trapped against the hand basin, and she ran out of the room.

At lunchtime we had a meeting with other members of the team. The atmosphere was terrible and I felt totally abandoned. Those who were my friends on the team felt unable to say anything to support me, for fear of alienating Dr and Mrs C. Of course I understood. They were going to have to continue working with them, and did not want to be the next victim of their bullying tactics. I understood, but it hurt. They needed the work; they needed the income; but, at that moment, I'm afraid I did feel they were really condoning what had happened to me, especially as they had all witnessed the unacceptable behaviour.

I have never felt as lonely as I felt that day. The loneliness of being branded the enemy was almost unbearable. It was certainly impossible to concentrate. I am sure my patient management was inadequate.

My last day at the dysfunctional practice

Living among scorpions

It is not a coincidence that up until now I have considered one day in particular both the best and worst day of my working life.

It was the beginning of the May half-term holiday.

I was not meant to be working that Tuesday, and planned to spend the day with my young daughters; I had been on call during the Bank Holiday Monday and overnight until Tuesday morning, covering two practices, and also police work. Just before the end of the shift, I had an urgent phone call from a palliative care patient, who needed hospital admission. I also had to phone the coroner regarding another patient who had died suddenly.

I left my daughters at home and drove to the surgery to complete these tasks. I was not expecting to be long. I knew I had one more surgery to work on Wednesday morning before leaving the practice, and all the animosity, behind me.

On arrival at the surgery, a locum was the only doctor conducting a surgery, so I tried to sort out the problems as quickly as possible. The palliative care patient was requesting admission to a private hospital, but as she was in a great deal of pain, it might have been wiser to go to accident and emergency.

Mrs C, the practice manager, arrived and I remembered that it was her birthday. Although I had been 'banned' from saying anything that might upset her, I was not prepared to be uncivil, so I greeted her by simply saying 'happy birthday'. She reacted by throwing the post all over the front counter and then barging into the room I was using, whilst I was on the phone.

She came right up to me and said 'that was completely unnecessary!'

She circled round me like a boxer. It felt very threatening. She had phoned her husband to come in so that he could sort me out. She ranted about how awful I was. Her behaviour was so out of control I threatened to call the police. Suddenly she said 'you tried to preach to me about Ezekiel chapter 2!' (I didn't realise the significance of this comment until later, but Ezekiel 2 describes God's calling of Ezekiel to be a prophet and to go to preach to the stubborn and rebellious Israelites. He was told to go and preach whether they listened or not; he was to be obedient to God.)

The following is an extract from the record I made at the time. (After every difficult encounter I would go home and write down the conversations as accurately as possible.)

Mrs C [shouting at the top of her voice]: Do your work and don't say anything to me tomorrow!
Hazel: If you are like this tomorrow, I will call the police.
Mrs C left the room and then re-entered.
Mrs C: I'm not frightened. (But she looked terrified and had phoned her husband to sort me out.)

At this point Dr C stormed into the practice building and into the room where I was working, which was his consulting room, and slammed the door shut.

This was a very frightening situation and I wasn't sure what would happen. He clearly had no intention of finding out if I was trying to manage a patient. The fact that this was a working general practice, and there was a very sick patient desperately waiting to be admitted to hospital, was irrelevant. He failed to ask me what work I was trying to do, all he was interested in was his practice, and as far as he was concerned, I was there to cause as much disruption as possible, and I had threatened the unthinkable – to involve the police.

Hazel: Dr C… please…

Dr C [interrupts, shouting at the top of his voice]: I haven't done anything yet!

This is my practice

This is my room

These are my patients

These are my staff

This is my job and this is my building

This is my room and in my room I can do whatever I like!

Hazel [In the heat of the moment but as calmly and quietly as possible!]: I'm very frightened. Your wife is out of control, and. two weeks ago she might even have run me over in the car park if I hadn't moved out of the way.

Dr C [angrily- but without questioning the validity of the accusation]: Quite frankly I'm surprised she hasn't shot you!

At this point he left the room and suggested to his wife that they went upstairs to calm down.

This was my lifeline. I was still trying to admit my patient, but I suddenly realised that I could continue the phone calls from her house. I had to leave the building before they came back downstairs.

The room I had been using and the reception area are quite dark. As I left the building I was dazzled by the brightness of the sun. A Christian healthcare assistant had just parked in the car park. She looked at me and asked if I was leaving. I explained I still had one more surgery to take, the following day. She replied with real insight, 'you don't want to do it, do you?' I shook my head and drove off.

As I was leaving one of my patients with her seventeen-year-old daughter walked past me and into the waiting room. They subsequently spoke to the practice manager, asking for appointments to see me. Triumphantly, she announced that I had left, and if they wanted to see me they would have to change practices. I know this because the girl subsequently became a friend of my daughters.

I drove to the cancer patient's house and used the phone in her bedroom to arrange the admission, and an ambulance. I asked her if I could phone my home to tell my daughters where I was. At that time I did not have my own mobile phone.

My younger daughter Rachel answered the phone and immediately I knew something was wrong. She said, 'Mummy, Dr C phoned; he phoned twice. He accused Marian of lying.' I asked her what she meant and she explained he asked her if mummy was at home, and on the second occasion, when she said 'no,' he didn't believe her.

I felt awful; I had left my children unprotected. I had exposed them to the wrath of my GP partner and his wife. I put the phone down and thought I was going to faint from the shock. The cancer patient was very caring, in spite of her pain, and confirmed to me, in what she said, how discreet I had actually been throughout the

Learning To Be (the) Patient

traumatic time. She asked 'Are you all right? Would you like me to call Dr C to come and look after you?'

I said that would not be necessary!

She had no idea that he was the cause of my distress, and as far as I know never did.

I waited until the ambulance arrived, but had to get home as quickly as possible. What if the phone rang again and Marian had to answer it again?

As soon as I got home I rang my husband, Nick, to come home as I didn't want to speak to Dr C either. When I phoned him at work he was furious that Dr C had involved our children in our dispute, and came home immediately.

Bearing in mind I was still due to work the following day, I wanted advice on how to stop Mrs C from interfering with my work. I was advised to see if I could obtain an injunction, but on speaking to a solicitor I realised I had left it too late.

My husband phoned Dr C. He demanded to speak to me, but Nick wouldn't let him. He asked him if he would tell his wife to stay away from the practice the following day, to leave me in peace, but he would not. So my husband asked him how he would guarantee my safety, but he could not, and rang off.

We decided we had two options: Nick would have to sit in the waiting room for the entire morning and, if necessary, we would call the police. I would let them know I might need them, first thing in the morning.

Dr C phoned back. Again, Nick answered. He had decided to take the surgery himself, and I was never to return to the practice.

As the patients were booked to see me I sought further advice and put in writing that he could see the patients, and I would return a keys, etc to him. My husband delivered the letter and went back to work. He made it absolutely clear that they were to have no contact with me.

My relief at knowing I didn't have to go back was huge, but I had one set of patient's notes with me and a very old practice dictaphone, to dictate a referral for this patient.

The doorbell rang and I realised it was Dr C. He had taken no notice of my husband's request not to have any contact, and had come round to my house within an hour of the conversation. Considering what he had said to me earlier, I had no idea what he would do, but did not want to leave him on the doorstep. I called the girls to stand on either side of me and, terrified, opened the door. He handed me the waste paper bin that I had left in the consulting room, and then angrily accused me of stealing the dictaphone. I explained I still had a letter to do, and one set of notes in my possession. This confused him. He stood in silence, uncertain what to say. Eventually, he decided to take the notes and the dictaphone, and dictate the letter himself.

I have never spoken to him again.

I took the girls to the cinema in the afternoon. It didn't matter what we saw, we needed to get away from the house and try to relax. I had put them through an ordeal to which they should never have been exposed.

Reflection on the events of the day

That evening I reflected on the strange comment Mrs C had made earlier that day: 'You tried to preach to us on Ezekiel 2.'

Months earlier I had told her a story that I had heard during a sermon whilst visiting our friends Alison and Chris, in Stockport. I was deeply upset at the time. It was the start of the troubles at the surgery. I had been pressured by Mrs C to buy into the practice, in other words to own part of the building. It had taken me six months to negotiate the loan and get to the point where contracts could be exchanged. I had had to work very hard, in my own time, to reach this point. Suddenly, Dr C decided he had never really decided to sell, and withdrew the offer. I was very upset. I felt rejected, even though he felt nothing had changed in our relationship as business partners.

They could not understand why I was hurt.

The story I recounted was a simple story which I naïvely hoped might help them understand why I was upset. The sermon covered Ezekiel chapter 2 and the beginning of chapter 3. (Ezekiel was called by God to speak to the rebellious Israelites but was warned he might be ignored – his message rejected.)

The story I heard during the sermon was about door-to-door salesmen. It went something like this. Apparently 'in the days of carbon-paper salesmen, there were too many salesmen and very little demand. People didn't want to buy. The average length of time they stayed in the job was six months. At the end of six months they felt totally rejected. They were equating rejection of the product with rejection of themselves. They had had enough of being rejected.' This story was used to illustrate a point made in Ezekiel chapter 3.

As I listened to the sermon a huge weight was lifted from my shoulders. It was all right to feel rejected; I wasn't overreacting. I had been working on a project for six months. It wasn't unreasonable for me to equate rejection of my commitment to buy a portion of the practice, with rejection of myself.

I wanted to try to get them to understand. I told Mrs C this story. In a difficult situation I often find it easier to tell a story to illustrate a point. At the time I mentioned that the sermon was on Ezekiel chapter 2 and 3, but then just told the story.

After my encounter with Mrs C on her birthday, I realised she must have read the chapters. This had not been my intention, and I could see why she was upset, but I'm afraid it really amused me. I realised she would have read a description of herself and maybe she worked this out.

Ezek. 2: 6: 'And you, son of man, be not afraid of them, nor be afraid of their words, though briers and thorns are with you and you sit upon scorpions; be not afraid of their words, nor be dismayed at their looks, for they are a rebellious house.'

I don't know if she did read this, but I know working with Mrs C was like working with a scorpion. So often when she said something there was a sting in its tail.

Reflection: the need to encourage rather than demoralise

It has taken me many years to realise quite how destructive Mrs C's behaviour was both to me and to my staff. She had made it very clear that when a person joined the staff she studied them to assess their faults. I had been shocked at this, and upset. The practice manager was not looking for people's gifts, to enhance the quality of their work, or to encourage and compliment them, but was looking for ways to criticise and demoralise them; something to sting them with when felt she was losing control. Her observation concerning me was that I didn't take my work seriously enough. I now realise that what she said to me, when she said that I didn't take my work seriously enough (implying that I laugh and smile too much), was worse than just focusing on a fault. She had identified a quality in me that patients and staff found helpful and had turned it into a fault. She was trying to destroy what was good. Likewise, if in conversation I had commented on how pleased I was with someone's work, the job was soon removed from them. Only the practice manager was allowed to 'shine' in that place.

Worse than just trying to destroy a helpful quality in me, she was actually trying to undermine an aspect of my consultation that can actually be the beginning of real healing: a light-hearted moment where previously there had only been despair; a rekindling of hope where previously there had been none.

Reflection on my behaviour

Was it inappropriate to greet Mrs C that morning with 'Happy birthday'? Was I deliberately trying to provoke her?

As I said, I had been 'banned' by Dr C from speaking to Mrs C, my employee, unless absolutely necessary, but I wanted to remain civil. The Christian principles I live by reflect my desire always to treat others as I would have them treat me. We were all meant to be part of a team. I still wanted to show respect to my partner and all my employees. This included my practice manager who was one of my employees, even though she behaved as if she were my boss, and I one of her slaves with whom she could do whatever she liked. To his credit Dr C always spoke civilly to me in front of patients and staff when I greeted him. He only became angry behind closed doors.

I have often questioned whether when I greeted Mrs C with 'good morning', or 'happy birthday' I was mimicking her behaviour. I perceived her tone as mocking, particularly when she asked me questions like 'where's your God now, is he talking to you?' after she had thrown something at me. She reacted as if my tone was also mocking when I greeted her. This was not intentional, and I certainly never threw anything at her, spat at her or became abusive. It took a great deal of courage to walk into surgery each day, and civilly greet both Dr and Mrs C, knowing that abuse might well follow, but my aim was to be courteous. I tried to demonstrate the meaning of 'showing respect' for everyone throughout my time there, even for those who considered themselves my enemies.

What appeared to be happening was a form of projection. Mrs C was interpreting whatever I said in the light of her feelings towards me. Because she appeared only to harbour hatred and anger towards me, she assumed that my attitude must be the same, and anything I said, however polite, was considered appalling. During this time I clung to my Christian faith, desperate to demonstrate love for my enemies, but really struggled as whatever I said made it worse.

I can honestly say that I longed for reconciliation, even if just to facilitate my leaving, but they appeared to have absolutely no insight into this at all.

My dream: reconciliation

Having a diagnosis of cancer certainly makes you focus on what's important. At the hospice we talk of 'unfinished business'; the things the patient still needs to sort out before they die. Reconciliation with estranged members of the family; the healing of broken relationships, is a high priority, and very powerful.

More than a decade later I would still love to sit down with Dr and Mrs C and talk it through, with a mediator, to resolve the conflict. Forgiveness is the Christian way and so much part of my life. It has been very hard living with the knowledge that this would probably never happen. I know how important it is to 'move on' leaving the past behind, and sometimes there is so much hurt it seems best buried; but there have been such fine examples, for example in South Africa, in recent years of where 'truth and reconciliation' has worked powerfully to build up, rather than destroy.

I was very concerned about Mrs C's mental state, in particular. She seemed so embittered. She seemed totally incapable of maintaining friendships once there had been any disagreement. She always had to make a fresh start with someone new, until that relationship soured. History had repeated itself over and over again. She seemed unable to learn from her mistakes. As well as being my employee and the wife of my GP partner, she was also registered with me as a patient. This was a serious error on my part, but she had been registered with the previous partner, and her registration was transferred to me on my arrival. I never saw her handwritten medical record. It was kept locked away, even from her own GP.

When I first joined the practice this seemed a relatively trivial matter, but as her mental state deteriorated, I became increasingly concerned for her as a patient who had branded her own GP her enemy, and needed psychological help, but, of course, could not ask for advice from me. It was unthinkable for her to seek my help; she had never sought medical advice from me, and during the dispute, when her need was greatest, a doctor/patient relationship was impossible. Although a true doctor/patient relationship was never possible, I am aware that as the relationship between us deteriorated, but before I was 'banned' from talking to her, I had several difficult conversations with her, on her own. These were not normal conversations between two colleagues. I would sit quietly, waiting for her to break the silence. I would wait patiently, knowing that she hated silence. I listened and observed her carefully waiting for her to make an irrational, insulting or paranoid comment. I had to concentrate to ensure I had really heard her correctly. Even with good psychiatric training, I have always found it difficult to accurately recall irrational remarks. When I talked to Mrs C I now realise I wasn't listening to her as a colleague, I was performing mental health assessments on her.

Of course this was all I could do; I could observe, but do no more. Her husband was the only person who could provide medical care, and it was impossible to discuss this with him. This was a very unsatisfactory situation. I considered asking her to leave the practice list and register elsewhere, which is recommended practice anyway, but I knew this would inflame the situation further. She was the practice manager and it was her job to sort out patient's transfers. She wasn't going to request her own compulsory removal from my list! My hands were completely tied. She was becoming sick and I was her doctor but she thought of me as her enemy.

I can understand why Mrs C considered me her enemy. Eventually, she became aware of the reason I had given for my resignation: I could not work with her any longer. She pinned up on her office wall the quotation: 'Hell hath no fury like a woman scorned.' For her this was a declaration of war, a war of verbal abuse on her part, but a legal battle on mine.

It would be wrong to claim that I was not tempted to play their games. I mentioned the quotation to my husband who pointed out that the quotation should read, 'Nor Hell a fury, like a woman scorn'd', but it is commonly misquoted. The idea of anonymously correcting the error on the piece of paper was very tempting, but I knew it would cause Mrs C great distress, provoking further insults. I had to minimise the effect her anger and bad behaviour had on other staff and patients.

Unfortunately for them, their bullying tactics were never going to be adequate. As long as I stood firm, and persevered I knew that legal advice was what I needed. As far as I know they never sought legal advice regarding the partnership dispute; however, he did phone the BMA adviser to tell him what he thought of him. I understand it was not a pleasant conversation.

My desire for conciliation following resignation

Once I had officially resigned from the partnership, I spoke to Dr C about my leaving terms. He was adamant that I needed to stick to the terms of the partnership agreement to work six months' notice. This was something I realised would probably be unbearable for everyone, not least the patients. I asked him if we could involve a conciliator who would help us look at things rationally. I was aware that this would not be comfortable for either of us but, at least, there would be an independent observer to try to ensure decisions were made fairly.

I asked him if he would be prepared to consider conciliation so that both our points of view would be taken into consideration, but he would not listen, and angrily dismissed the whole idea. At this point I knew I would never achieve anything through discussion on my own with him, but it was impossible to persuade him to involve anyone else. If Dr C had accepted the help of the BMA conciliator, and we had been able to comply with the terms, patient care would have been less compromised.

Instead of a face-to-face discussion guided by a conciliator, I needed to put the hard facts in writing. I knew that the facts, spelt out in a carefully drafted letter, would cause great distress, because even though I had tried to express my feelings and concerns, they had not been listened to. With the aid of the BMA adviser, we managed to demonstrate that Dr C had breached the partnership agreement within days of us signing it, so I wasn't under obligation to comply with it either. This meant I eventually informed them formally, in writing, that I would only work three months' notice, rather than the six months stated in the partnership agreement. The Cs were extremely angry as they accused me of 'leaving them in the lurch' and losing the practice money in locum fees, but this might have been averted if Dr C had understood the rationale behind conciliation.

Each evening after a difficult conversation with either Dr or Mrs C, I wrote down as much of the conversation as I could recall, whilst it was still fresh in my mind.

I have now reread the transcript of the conversation that I had had with Dr C regarding the use of conciliation, after he had received the letter telling him I would only work three months' notice, and clearly spelling out the reasons why.

I was quite shocked when I reread it to see how illogical and weak Dr C's arguments were. He only really had one argument, which he repeated over and over again, whilst becoming increasingly angry. The following is an extract demonstrating that he would never consider involvement of a third party, even though he complained that no one had heard his point of view.

He had received the letter, drafted by my advisers, saying I would be leaving at the end of May, rather than August, as he had breached the partnership agreement.

Dr C: You can leave when I appoint another partner; you will be breaking the partnership agreement if you go at the end of May, and I will sue you.

Hazel: Yes but you are already in breach of the partnership agreement... it's in my letter, clearly stated.

Dr C: It's not in your letter.

Hazel: Yes it is [producing a copy of the letter].

Dr C: That letter is evil; it's the most evil thing I have ever been sent. It's full of lies.

Hazel [quoting an excerpt from the professionally drafted letter]: 'You allowed me no say in the decision to appoint Mrs C as practice manager. [You simply told me she was coming back and that she would be in the post until you retire.] This is not in accordance with section... of our partnership agreement. This says 'No member of staff can be appointed without the prior consent of both partners'.

Dr C: You left it very late to bring this up!

Hazel: Yes, but you gave me no choice. I didn't want to bring it up like this – that's why I wanted to go to conciliation.

Dr C: You are the most ungrateful bitch. Conciliation, you are obsessed with conciliation – you're the only one who wants it.

Dr C: The letter's a pack of lies.

Hazel: It isn't a pack of lies. I remember the conversation on 1 March last year very clearly. You told me that our old practice manager was going to have to leave. I sat in silence for some time and then said, 'so what next?' You said your wife would be coming back as practice manager, and I asked if it would be temporary whilst we appointed someone else, but you said she would be practice manager until you retired. I had no choice, I only agreed after you had given me no choice. Then I told you I would not even have applied for the job if there had been a husband and wife team in place at the time.

Dr C: Yes, and you have said that since too [repeating himself]. The letter is the most evil thing I have received. You are the most unchristian Christian I know.

Hazel: I don't want to argue any further. I want someone else to be present.

Dr C: Oh we are going to have an argument…. About your Christian hypocrisy… the lies you told …..

Dr C [repeating himself]: Your letter was evil – I have shown it to someone already. I will keep it and show it to others as well.

Hazel: Who?

Dr C: [No response]

Hazel: I had professional help with my letter from two people who act as conciliators.

Dr C: Conciliators, they aren't conciliators, they only heard your side of the story.

Hazel: That's because you wouldn't let a conciliator hear your side!

Dr C [getting up to leave and returning to his original argument]: If you leave before the beginning of September you will be in breach of your partnership agreement.

Hazel: I *will* leave at the end of May, or beginning of June [so he could take his annual leave].

Dr C: I *will* sue you [walking out shutting the door].

Dr C [opening door and shouting]: *I hope you rot in hell* [slamming door shut].

Dr C [opening door again]: *You will rot in hell* [slamming door shut].

Dr C [opening door again]: But since you are still a partner you can lock up! [He left the building.]

I had tried so hard to have a reasoned discussion with him but I had failed. I knew the situation could only get worse. I will never know if a conciliator would have made a difference.

Arguments and counterarguments

The letter I gave to Dr C, stating that either I would leave at the end of May unless he was prepared to discuss things with the aid of a conciliator, read as follows:

Dear (Dr C),
Further to our conversation last Tuesday I write to inform you I wish to leave the practice as soon as my minimum three months' notice to the Buckinghamshire Health Board expires, ie at the end of May.

The situation at the surgery has become very difficult. The atmosphere is poor and five months is far too long for everyone to endure this. It is unsettling for the staff and is bound to have an adverse effect on the patients' perception of the practice. Despite our differences I do not want this to happen.

At present I am in the position where I, as a partner, am joint employer of the practice manager and therefore responsible for her actions and yet you have ordered me not to speak to her on practice matters.

This is an impossible situation and I am not prepared to work under these conditions. I recognise that our partnership agreement provides for a longer period of notice but I would point out that the present situation has arisen because you have breached both the spirit and the letter of the agreement.

In particular you allowed me no say in the decision to appoint (Mrs C) as practice manager (you simply told me that she would be in post until you retire). This is not in accordance with section 12.2.10 of our partnership agreement.

I have requested on at least three occasions that our dispute (in particular with regard to the practice manager) should be taken to arbitration or that we should ask an outside conciliator to help us talk things through. You have refused to consider this despite the provision of section 25 of our partnership agreement.

If you are not prepared to consider this further I feel I have no alternative but to leave as soon as possible which from my contract with Bucks Health Board is the end of May.

Yours, etc

I asked Dr C to respond in writing but he refused to do so saying that he would talk to me about it when he was ready, but again refused to talk to me with an independent observer present. He said he needed time to think it over, which I respected, and eventually told me he would talk to me about it at the end of evening surgery, after he had had a few days' leave.

The conversation was written down the same evening and is as accurate as possible and recorded in the section on 'my desire for conciliation following resignation'.

After evening surgery I went into his room to discuss the letter. He did not have it with him. He immediately gave me the only reply he was going to give me.

Dr C: You can leave when I appoint another partner, you will be breaking the partnership agreement if you go at the end of May and I will sue you.

I briefly established that he had not got anyone in mind and there were no new applicants, so it was highly unlikely that a new partner would be appointed before September, so he wasn't in fact even offering me a compromise. The emphasis was on the 'I will sue you'. The aim was to try to frighten me into submission. He was making it clear that he was in charge, he was the boss and I was to do what he said, or there would be severe repercussions. I had already come to realise that he viewed the partnership agreement as a contract that he expected me to obey, but with no acknowledgement that he should adhere to it as well. It was his practice and he was in control.

My reply to his opening statement tried to focus on the content of my letter, and to point out that I knew that I would be breaking the agreement, but the letter had fully addressed the issue.

Hazel: Yes but you are already in breach of the partnership agreement… it's in my letter, clearly stated.

Dr C: It's not in your letter.

This was his immediate reply. He did not have the letter with him, or at least did not produce it at any stage during the conversation, but did he really think I would not have a copy with me? His tone of voice was becoming more aggressive. As he had had days to read the letter and seek legal advice, if he had wanted to, I did not believe he had failed to understand the letter, but again was trying to get me to retract my comments and submit to his orders.

When I produced a copy of the letter his attitude became even more unpleasant. As he was clearly unable to produce a reasoned counterargument to the content of my letter, the discussion became nasty.

Dr C: That letter is evil; it's the most evil thing I have ever been sent. It's full of lies.

Again, I felt he was just trying to frighten me. On several occasions I had tried to raise the issues mentioned in the letter with him, but I knew he wasn't listening. Seeing it in writing must have been a shock. I wanted to avoid this scenario, but he hadn't co-operated, so in the end I had had to write it down. Seeing it written down in black and white meant he couldn't ignore what was there, but he was still trying to. Initially, he tried to pretend it wasn't in the letter at all, but when confronted with a copy, he chose to accuse me of lying and doing evil.

He had breached the partnership agreement within days of us signing it, by forcing the resignation of the practice manager, and reinstating his wife, without allowing me any say in the matter. My legal advisers made it clear that the partnership agreement was, therefore, no longer valid. I wanted to discuss this with him face to face, with the help of the legal adviser acting as conciliator. As Dr C had refused repeatedly to involve a third party, the breach of the agreement had to be put in writing. He was not aware of this argument until he received the letter. I was aware that it would be difficult, and warned him that the content would be hard to read, when I handed him the letter.

When I explained to him that I hadn't wanted him to 'just see it in writing' but to 'hear it in the presence of a conciliator' he became more abusive, calling me a 'most ungrateful bitch'.

It was this type of insult I was trying to avoid, by requesting the presence of an independent observer. I had experienced this sort of language before, in previous discussions, and had had enough of his unprofessional attitude.

Returning to the subject of the letter, he repeated his argument that the letter was 'a pack of lies'.

This led me to quietly remind him of the conversation we had had at the time of the forced resignation of the practice manager.

Hazel: You told me our old practice manager was going to have to leave...'

He agreed that the conversation had taken place but still insisted that the letter was evil (but no longer a 'pack of lies'). He chose instead to become more abusive, challenging my Christian faith instead, by accusing me of being the 'most unchristian Christian I know'.

He did not explain what he meant by this, but I assumed he thought that I should be meek and mild, and keep turning the other cheek whatever was thrown at me. He hadn't expected me to challenge them, and certainly not challenge their integrity.

As his language was starting to become more abusive, and I knew the conversation was going nowhere, I said I didn't want to argue any further, and requested that we only continue in the presence of a third party. He wasn't going to stop shouting at me, and became more and more abusive, accusing me of 'Christian hypocrisy'.

I knew the context of this. He was referring to an occasion a month earlier when Mrs C had hurriedly produced a new practice leaflet. The grammar was poor and there were spelling mistakes. No-one had been asked to proofread it and we were all embarrassed about it. One of the members of staff was very angry indeed about the way she had altered the front cover design, but no-one was prepared to speak to her about it, so I said that I would do it during our weekly business meeting. Mrs C was furious, especially when I said I wasn't the only one who was concerned. She immediately went to interrogate the members of staff, who of course modified their story. Of course they did; they didn't want to lose their jobs, and Mrs C's bullying tactics were extremely unpleasant. Inevitably, this was conclusive evidence that I had lied, and it was at this point that I was banned from speaking to Mrs C, and *all further weekly business meetings were cancelled even though I was meant to be working there for a further five months.*

Over time I had forgotten why I had been banned from speaking to Mrs C. I only remembered recently on rereading the notes I made at that time. It seems unbelievable now that she was so upset over me asking her to correct some simple spelling mistakes, but this happened and I was banned from speaking to her (except to be civil) in case I upset her again.

Complaints

During my last few weeks at the surgery the atmosphere was so tense, and the level of stress so high, that mistakes were bound to happen.

On one occasion a patient came into my room, apparently for a consultation, sat down and ordered me to record what he was about to say in the handwritten notes. He was very intimidating; I was being bullied by a patient now, whilst also being bullied by my colleagues. Of course, the patient knew there was no way he could make a complaint, about Dr C in a civilised way, by talking to the practice manager, so had decided to speak to me instead. He believed he had been given a drug he had already reported had caused him an adverse reaction. I believe, in retrospect, it was a trivial reaction.

The week before I resigned I had been on holiday with my daughters. On my return Dr C asked me to see him in his consulting room, after morning surgery. He had a pile of patient notes on his desk. I knew what was about to happen; he had done this before. It was a selection of notes from patients I had seen in the previous few weeks. He had found the record in the notes that the patient had bullied me into writing. He was furious, and had decided to take revenge, and find fault with as many consultations as possible. He did not listen to my explanation that I had been bullied by the patient, and told me the patient had lied to me. The reason he was furious was that, obviously, he would now be 'throwing' the patient off his list, so when he registered at another practice, another doctor would read the note, and it would affect Dr C's reputation. I'm afraid that what the patient may have gossiped to his neighbours was likely to be more damaging.

In his interrogation of me he demanded to know why I had labelled a young boy as 'allergic to penicillin', accusing me of inappropriate diagnosis. I explained that he had had a severe rash whilst on the drug, to which he replied I hadn't emphasised the severity adequately. He clearly wanted to make me feel very uncomfortable. I was told by members of staff that both Dr and Mrs C had been involved in the process of finding as many sets of notes with potential errors in as possible. The atmosphere had been very tense whilst I was away, and they had witnessed the behaviour before.

After each accusation he slammed the notes down and opened the next. The final and, as far as he was concerned, worst fault, was my completion of an insurance medical report. The patient had been to see Dr C because the insurance premium had been 'loaded' due to one significant disorder. He accused me of being 'too honest' on the form and not being supportive enough of the patient. At the end of the very unpleasant bullying session I realised the main accusation he had against me was that I was being too honest!

He was telling me off for telling the truth. Was he really telling me he wanted me to be deceitful? I felt he was asking me to leave because I had told the truth!

I asked him if he was hoping I would resign but he denied this.

On my return from my holiday he certainly had not made any effort to welcome me back or convince me he still wanted to work with me. I was very concerned about his accusation that I was too honest. How could honesty be a vice in his eyes?

A week later, after I had resigned, I received a letter from another insurance company, concerning another patient. This was a medical report that had been sent to me to complete whilst I was away. Dr C had filled it in instead and sent it to the company. Their medical officer had written to me asking me why I had omitted an important and potentially serious diagnosis from the report. They already knew about the diagnosis because the patient had declared it herself. I was informed that potentially I could be charged with fraud for failing to list significant diagnoses.

I already knew this, but it reassured me that honesty was essential when completing these forms. As my relationship with Dr C had completely broken down I did not feel able to mention it to him, and certainly did not want him to reply to the insurance company. I completed a further form for them, including the significant diagnosis, and sent it back. Fortunately, this was accepted by them and legal proceedings were avoided. I wondered if this was the first time he had deliberately left a diagnosis off a medical report to save the patient money, or how he would have reacted if he had seen the letter from the company. I feared he might well have lost his temper and rung the company doctor to give him an 'earful'.

Giving patients an earful was something I discovered by chance happened on a fairly regular basis, when I met a patient who had chosen to move to another practice. As she had changed practices we had received a request for her notes from the health authority. Mrs C had seen the list, noted that the patient had not moved away from the area, so had passed her name to Dr C to ring her up and find out why she had moved. According to the patient he had ranted over the phone, accusing her of being disloyal and demanding to know why she had left. His attitude over the phone confirmed to her that she had made the right decision. I was extremely embarrassed about his behaviour especially because on asking the Cs about this, I discovered they considered this normal practice, something that he had done for years when patients changed practices in the area. It definitely ensured they never tried to move back again!

Later, after I left I met the mother of a girl who had survived a very serious illness and was expecting a visit from Dr C. She rang the surgery asking why he hadn't visited. When he did visit he was stressed and angry. Communication between the mother and Dr C was poor. She told me he did not accept he had failed in any way (and maybe he hadn't) but his attitude was appalling. In fact, he told her that his longstanding older patients considered him to be 'god'. In other words: 'How dare you question me'?

After I left, I know he became increasingly stressed and tired as he had to do extra on-call sessions, but his arrogance clearly upset this girl's mother. I am uncertain how communication had broken down between the family and the practice, but in the middle of all the arguments was a young girl who had nearly died, who needed to be able to trust the medical profession for her future care.

I was branded completely unsupportable when the practice finally had two complaints against me. Mrs C had been longing to receive a complaint about me, and had been doing her best to provoke me into making a mistake by disrupting my surgeries. The first complaint came from a patient for whom I had prescribed the antibiotic trimethoprim. He mentioned to the nurse that it gave him 'thrush' but, as it was the most appropriate antibiotic I advised, he should take it anyway, and we would treat the thrush, particularly as many antibiotics can do this. Unfortunately 'thrush' turned out to be an allergic reaction.

I don't know what Mrs C said to the patient but I never had the opportunity to speak to him or apologise. She triumphantly told me how appalling I was and that I was 'on my own' if the complaint went further – I was completely unsupportable.

The other complaint was from an angry mother of a toddler who needed referral. I understand she complained to the practice manager about me. I referred him to the local hospital that then transferred his care to London. At this point she saw my original referral letter, and was angry. On one occasion the mother had appeared intoxicated on attending the surgery and I had tried to warn my colleagues.

Again, I do not know how the complaint was handled by Mrs C, but I was given to understand I would be hearing from the General Medical Council. I heard nothing at all, but met the patient sometime later in the supermarket. She was friendly, chatty and proud of the fact she had turned her life round.

Either Mrs C had managed the complaint better than I feared she had, or she had made it sound far worse than it was, to make me feel as uncomfortable as possible.

Unacceptable revenge

I left the practice on 30 May but did not move from the area. Despite Mrs C's declaration that once other professionals heard what I had done I would never get another job, I have not, in fact, been out of work at all. Now that I am on sick leave this is my first extended period off work since. I needed to keep busy to try to prove to myself I was good enough, and I was fit to work.

Slowly over time, as I met patients at the shops or met members of staff socially, I learnt what happened after I left.

Because I had been 'ordered' by Dr and Mrs C not to tell people that I was leaving, I had to make sure no one discussed it in the waiting room. I realised that the ban by the Cs was totally inappropriate. How could I maintain patients' trust in my management and care without explaining I was leaving? The Cs wanted to make it look as if they had thrown me out, yet I had worked my notice, and I wanted to say 'goodbye' and ensure appropriate follow-up. I wanted to ensure that they understood the plan for their future management. It would have been so irresponsible of me not to tell my patients I was about to leave. I told specific patients discreetly, without going into detail, but had to tell them not to talk about it, which, of course made them suspicious. The patients were not stupid; they had observed the departure of previous female doctors from the practice, and some had observed the behaviour of Mrs C in other social situations, and guessed relationship problems were the underlying cause.

I tried to leave adequate notes on the patients, but I was not allowed to talk to any locum successor and of course it was impossible to talk to Dr C. Patient care was compromised.

On the day I left Dr and Mrs C took a black bin bag into my consulting room and stripped it of everything that reminded them of me. They also changed the burglar alarm code and placed a tatty handwritten notice in the waiting room informing the patients that 'Dr Butland has left the practice'. There were no words of regret or apology. They were obviously delighted. I heard that patients who asked why I had left were told they got rid of me because I was 'too religious'. I had certainly challenged the ethics of their practice.

Obviously, as I had left they had had the last word. I just had to trust that patients who had got to know me over the twenty months would realise that I was trying to work with integrity, and had wanted to do the best for them all.

There were several incidents that made me angry and very concerned about the practice, following my departure.

I discovered that other members of staff had actually resigned and left after they had been badly treated by the practice manager.

No post was ever forwarded to me. If any patient wrote to me expressing regret that I had left, I never saw it, but I knew this would be the case. More worryingly, some hospital letters and laboratory results which I had requested, were sent to their surgery whilst I was working as a locum elsewhere, but I never received them. Patient care may have been compromised in this situation, but it wasn't a police matter. Unfortunately, the following incident was.

I was still working as a police surgeon up until the day I left. Although it did not occur very often, the police occasionally wrote to me at the surgery to request a statement, regarding a prisoner, due to appear in court. The statements are always needed urgently. When the police officer contacted the surgery to find out why the statement had not been written, he was informed I had left the practice, and subsequently told me he was advised I had moved to Scotland. Fortunately, he thought to try my 'old' home address and was surprised to find me still there. I was shocked when I realised that Mrs C was even happy to lie to the police, even though Dr C was still working as a police surgeon himself.

Another incident made me far angrier as it involved a lovely, but vulnerable patient. I had got to know her well and used to visit her at home. We discussed many things, including our shared spiritual beliefs. Mrs C decided to befriend her as well as she was a neighbour.

Just before I left, I wanted to tell this lady that I was leaving, and say goodbye. I knew she would be upset and I was too. I had to go to visit her and parked near the house. Mrs C must have driven past the house whilst I was visiting and spotted the car, and guessed I was visiting her. She established that the patient had not requested a visit and was furious with me.

Writing this, years later, it seems unbelievable that this was considered unacceptable behaviour by the practice manager. There was absolutely no reason why I couldn't choose to visit a sick patient without her requesting a visit, but during this stressful time I had learnt to anticipate this type of accusation, and this level of paranoia. I always had to keep 'one step ahead'.

I subsequently heard from the patient again; she told me that after I left the practice Mrs C had done her very best to ridicule her faith. This was a woman who had been facing up to the possibility of sudden death and Mrs C had deliberately sought to destroy her faith, almost certainly to undermine her trust in me. What sort of person tries to remove the one hope that this patient had – that if she did die next week she had the hope of eternal life? What was driving this woman to interfere like this? How many other patients suffered at her hands? I will never know but it was a great relief when she finally embarked on another career completely outside the caring professions.

Makarios

Why am I writing all this?

For whom am I writing it? What is the purpose?

This must not be written so it reads, 'Look what I went through, aren't I marvellous?' but written in such a way that the reality of the situation is conveyed. My desire is to write this to reflect the nature of the Christian life, and to reflect on the discipline needed to 'run the race'. I also want to highlight the joy that seems unbelievable, unless you have felt it, of experiencing the overwhelming love of God when you reach 'rock bottom', and don't feel you can endure any more; suddenly in the midst of the storm there is the most amazing feeling of love and security. You can do no more; you are totally dependant on God to protect you.

I am writing this now because I am aware I am suffering again, but this time because I have breast cancer. It has helped me to reflect, and focused my mind, as I do not know how much time I have left.

I do not know who else will read this, but I am writing this for my daughters, so they understand what they had to endure as children, and to encourage them, at the beginning of their careers, to hold fast to their Christian principles, and to trust God, knowing that no matter what they are going through He will be with them. 'Even though I walk through the valley of the shadow of death, I fear no evil, for thou art with me.'

In recent years, far too much emphasis has been put on the wonders of the Christian life, linking it to prosperity and happiness, but so often ignoring the massage of suffering, even though this is clearly illustrated over and over again, first in the life and death of Jesus, and subsequently in the life of St Paul and the other apostles.

During the traumatic last few months at this dysfunctional practice, I was unable to reflect deeply on what was going on. I needed to be totally focused on the job in hand, to anticipate what might happen next, to cope with the next shower of abusive language. It has taken more than a decade, a philosophy and ethics course, and a diagnosis of breast cancer, to slow me down sufficiently to reflect properly on the experience, and it took several years to hear the words I longed to hear, from the moment I walked out of the building for the last time.

I was sitting in the big top, at the beginning of Spring Harvest 2000, at Easter, and the speaker was talking about the Beatitudes at the beginning of the Sermon on the Mount (Matt. 5: 3-12: Blessed are the poor in spirit, for theirs is the kingdom of heaven etc). What he then said was so profound, I don't know if I took in any more of the talk, but what he said was what I had been waiting to hear for years. Maybe I would have heard it before, if I hadn't been so busy working, and chasing around after my daughters, but I think I needed it shouted out loud. The speaker explained that although the Beatitudes are usually translated 'Happy are' or 'blessed are' the best translation of the phrase makarioi oi *is 'congratulations' or 'well done!' All of a sudden I had heard what I had longed to hear – something I could have heard years ago if it hadn't been lost in translation:*

Matt 5: 11: Congratulations to you when men revile you and persecute you and utter all kinds of evil against you falsely on my account. Rejoice and be glad, for your reward is great in heaven.

I had longed to hear 'well done' or 'congratulations' and at last I had.

Throughout the last few months at that surgery, the thing that had kept me going was the firm belief that I was being obedient to God. I had felt when I accepted the post that I had been called to work there, but hadn't anticipated what would happen. However, very shortly after starting the job, I discovered a significant unmet need that I was equipped to manage. I met some very needy and profoundly depressed Christian patients who needed very sensitive support and care. Through these people the Lord made it very clear that he wanted me there. It is such a joy to see them now, to have fellowship with them from time to time, and see how the Lord healed and restored them, to see their lives flourishing again; and I helped, in a small way all those years ago.

I believe the Lord confirmed my calling very clearly four to five months before I left. This was perfect timing, as I wouldn't have taken the job if I had seen the passage as a clear message for me at the beginning.

I had driven up to Manchester to stay with Chris and Alison and visit our friend who was dying of cancer. I was extremely upset at the time, and really struggling to sleep, so the long drive was probably dangerous; at least it got me away from home and helped me to think more rationally. Going to church with Alison and Chris was refreshing and I could really listen and take in the sermon. The sermon was so special, and so important; it was as if it had been written solely with me in mind. Chris and Alison were aware of my situation and felt the same.

The week before I travelled to Manchester Dr C had finally decided that he didn't want me to purchase a share of the practice, saying that he had never actually made up his mind to sell. However, he still wanted me as a partner, and believed it made no difference to our working relationship; nothing had changed. This was his point of view, and neither he nor his wife could see that my point of view might be different.

It had taken me six months of hard work and negotiation, all in my own spare time, to reach the point where I had the funding to purchase a share the practice. I had managed to obtain a loan for many *thousands of pounds, but the goalposts had been moved so many times it had become increasingly stressful. The final complication arose when we had to redraft our practice agreement to have us as joint owners. The solicitors produced the new draft but, unfortunately, due to a typing error, omitted one part of a clause stating that we should both have our own personal accountants. Clearly to me, and the solicitors, this was a simple error in the 'first draft' of the agreement that could easily be rectified.*

The doctor and his wife, the practice manager, interpreted this completely differently. This was the solicitor saying that we could not have our own accountant! Mrs C phoned me at home. It was an extremely difficult phone call. It was impossible to reason with her. Much of what she said was an incoherent rant. In the end I had to put the phone down, as we were getting nowhere. It was becoming clearer to me that she was exhibiting significant paranoid ideation. I could not reason with her; there was absolutely no way she would believe it was a simple error. I am not sure if Dr C shared her delusional belief, but the level of stress at home must have been awful. As a result of this simple typing error, he said what he said, and decided to reject my offer to buy a share of the premises, saying he had never definitely decided to sell.

Ultimately, when I look back, my resignation was triggered by a simple typing error, completely irrationally misinterpreted by the practice manager, and accepted as such by her husband. I now see that I was rescued from a totally unacceptable situation by a very timely typing error! If I had bought into the practice it would have been far more difficult to extract myself from it, but as the next few months would show, the manager practised very unethically.

I was angry, hurt, confused and felt rejected. It had been the practice manager who had pushed me to get on and sort out the loan six months earlier, in the presence of the practice accountant, who witnessed Dr C's decision to sell; but at the time no minutes were taken, and nothing was put down in writing, and there was no written agreement. I felt he was lying but was also aware that his wife had put pressure on me, so had probably put huge pressure on him as well, so he may well have agreed to keep her quiet. Home life at times must have been extremely difficult for him, as she certainly didn't stop thinking about work when she left the premises, as her rant down the phone to me had highlighted. Home life must have also been very difficult for their three teenage boys when their mother was so out of control.

Finally

It has certainly taken me a long time to write up this account. I have put my thoughts and feelings down on paper rather than providing a systematic account. I hope that some of the issues discussed can be used constructively for teaching about an ethical approach to running a business.

Prior to publication of this journal, I wrote to Dr C giving him the opportunity to view the account, and giving him the right to reply. I enclosed a stamped addressed envelope. He did not reply.

The content of the letter was as follows:

1 October 2007

Dear (Dr C)

I hope you are well.

I am writing to let you know that over the last year I have been on extended sick leave whilst undergoing surgery, chemotherapy and radiotherapy. It has not been an easy time for me or my family, but I found that I could cope by keeping a journal of my cancer journey. It is a mixture of narrative and reflection. At times during my treatment my thoughts also turned back to the last weeks of my time at ... surgery. I included these reflections in my journal.

I am telling you this because I am planning to publish the journal. Those who have read the first draft have found it very helpful. I have not identified the surgery and neither you nor [Mrs C] is mentioned by name.

Just before I was diagnosed with cancer I had completed a postgraduate diploma on philosophy and medical ethics. It has been constructive to re-examine the situation with a greater understanding of that subject.

Obviously my journal is my story, so does not, at present, have your viewpoint. If you would like to read the relevant extracts prior to publication I would be happy to send them to you. Please include an alternative mailing address, if necessary.

I enclose a stamped addressed envelope for your initial response. If I haven't heard from you by the beginning of November I will assume it is OK to go ahead and publish.

Please understand I would be very happy to publish your reply and your side of the story.

I will include a copy of this letter (with names removed) at the end of the journal.

Yours sincerely, etc

Journal
March 2007 continued

Monday 19 March

I'm ten pounds lighter than this time last week in spite of another course of high-dose dexamethasone. Is 20 mg furosemide really this potent when you're not used to it?

My nails are changing; some are more affected than others. I think the growth has slowed down and they are very ridged now. I've been getting some right-sided rib pain as well, but I think this may just be pressure from my bra because of the fluid under the scar.

I had a wonderful surprise yesterday for Mothering Sunday. I got up late, and was about to have a shower before going to church, when Nick said very forcefully that he strongly recommended that I plan to attend the evening service, but not the morning service. I had no idea why, but then had a bath and took too long. At 10.30 a.m. as I was getting dressed, the front door opened very slowly and in walked Marian with a beautiful bunch of tulips. Everyone else knew she was coming but somehow they had managed to keep it a surprise. No wonder Nick had been behaving bizarrely when we were shopping on Saturday, making sure I bought too many vegetables and fruit. Unfortunately, I was so tired when we were shopping, I really wasn't in the mood for his jollity and longed for him to take note of my body language, and get home quickly. After all, I was only three days post-chemo, and it is really taking its toll now.

Yesterday, Laurence our vicar announced that he will be moving to look after some of the village churches in Buckinghamshire. This is not a great surprise but not what I wanted to hear just at the moment. I have gained so much from their support.

Wednesday 21 March

It's the first day of spring today. The sun is shining but it is cold outside! Two red kites soared over the house, really low this morning – what a beautiful sight.

I would like to try to go for a walk this afternoon, but I am so weak. I fell over on Sunday! I was crouching low down looking for a pack of blueberries in the fridge and I couldn't get up again. I toppled over backwards onto my bottom. Marian was quite concerned about my weakness. Most of the time I can use a chair, or some other item of furniture, to gain my balance and pull myself back up, but not this time.

Last night, my left hand and upper arm ached after doing my mosaic in day hospice. I certainly found it hard work cutting the tiles, even though they were soft ones. I am so pleased with what I am doing; it is so therapeutic!

I definitely feel like an old lady at the moment! I'm dithering as well. Time seems to be passing really slowly, and all I can really get my head round is when I can justify going back to bed for my afternoon nap. If I go too early I may not actually fall asleep, but if I leave it too late Nick may well wake me up when he comes in, which is not ideal.

I can't make up my mind what I should be doing, what I have the energy for and what is most important. I probably need to start keeping better lists of what needs to be done. My memory isn't good and I'm struggling to sound anything like articulate on the phone. It's really difficult to sound business-like! If I go upstairs, and then fail to remember why I went up, or just fail to do what I had intended, I can't just leap up and go up again; that's far too much for me at the moment. Going anywhere, even upstairs, needs a lot of planning. That sounds so pathetic, but it is so significant.

Sunday 25 March

Well I've got to Sunday and have neglected my journal!

Friday and Saturday were incredibly busy. I know I did too much, but I had committed myself to doing several things without thinking first about how I might be feeling. You would have thought I would have learnt by now, after all I have been having chemo since October last year. However, when I arranged the events I hadn't experienced the level of breathlessness or swelling of my legs that I have recently been getting.

Thursday evening we had the practice Christmas party! The food was reasonable but not fantastic. It would have been nice to have fresh vegetables rather than chips and peas! I didn't realise that we were going to have crackers, even though it is March. I amused those on our table by announcing to them all that my cracker contained a comb for my hair! Some of my hair is growing – in fact I never lost it completely – but it is just very thin on top. It's very grey at present, but in the mirror actually looks quite a lot nicer from the back since I had it trimmed. I still haven't got much hair anywhere else!

Late Friday afternoon, I went up to London and met Marian at Covent Garden. We had jacket potatoes in a little café, and then met up with her friends and their mothers to see *The Tempest* at the Novello theatre, with Patrick Stewart playing Prospero. I really enjoyed it, but we all agreed we preferred Marian's interpretation of Miranda. I do hope she gets a decent Shakespearian role to play this summer. I had to keep reminding Marian to slow down; although Covent Garden is the nearest tube to the theatre, it seemed a very long way! I travelled back very late by train and realised my ankles were beginning to swell again. I sat on the train with my legs on the seat, with my feet sticking off the end.

I got up very early on Saturday morning to catch the coach back up to London with Rachel, who had arrived home Friday evening to go to 'New Wine Women'. We met my friend Sheila up there, and I was really pleased as she thoroughly enjoyed it. My legs became very swollen and uncomfortable sitting in the seats and on the bus. I started to worry about developing a deep vein thrombosis. It would have been awful if I had been on an aeroplane! I was aware that although I was drinking enough I wasn't passing much urine. When we got home I realised how swollen I was again, and how much weight I had put on (six pounds). I took another furosemide 20 mg tablet, and after resting on the settee, went to bed early. I woke up several times during the night. My toes were burning and feet aching. Resting them on a pillow helped, but I struggled to get back to sleep. I wondered whether to take a sleeping tablet but decided not to, but eventually took an ibuprofen. I know that ibuprofen can cause further fluid retention, but I wanted some pain relief. In fact it worked well.

My wrists and hands feel swollen at present; they feel tight but my legs are more comfortable following the diuretic. Yesterday, at the day conference at Westminster Central Hall, we had several flights of stairs to climb. I managed them quite well the first time, but after lunch I was struggling to even climb the first flight. I was breathless and my pulse was racing. It is not a pleasant symptom at all. I would not have got up to the gallery a second time.

Psychological reflection

Just before I dropped to sleep during my afternoon siesta, I was inspired to produce a psychological reflection. I had a great idea! When I have a great idea I need to make a note of it immediately, otherwise I completely forget what it was. That is one of my problems at the moment. I will blame it on the chemotherapy, and general tiredness may be the cause, but my memory is deteriorating. I have also noticed my spelling is becoming more dyslexic and there are times when I am really struggling to read coherently. Yesterday, I was trying to read part of psalm 22 to Rachel and the words seemed all jumbled up. It was as if I had gone back to my childhood days when I really struggled to read out loud. It was so embarrassing and humiliating.

I had to stop, tell myself to concentrate and focus and then it was OK.

On Thursday I had lunch with an old friend Denise who works as a clinical psychologist in the chemotherapy unit at Stoke Mandeville, so it was partly therapeutic, and partly catching up!

Coping strategies: We talked about the fact I had been writing this journal and how writing it is therapeutic in itself. I know that it is one of my coping strategies. I am aware that when I wrote my dissertation, I wrote up some of the cases as a means of expressing my distress or anger. Again, that was very therapeutic. Denise asked me if the journal would need much editing; were there bits that I would feel were too embarrassing or sensitive to make public? I said I hadn't looked at it again yet, but I would not want to edit too much, as I might lose the impact of how I felt, and recorded it at the time. After all, feelings are modified over time, and it was important to capture my initial thoughts and feelings, especially when the news was bad.

Tuesday 27 March

I am really struggling with my legs this evening. They are so swollen and I have put even more weight on in spite of taking a furosemide tablet this morning. My weight is back up to eleven stone six pounds and I am breathless again. My legs feel so heavy to lift and my arms feel tight. My face is puffy and my hands are puffy. I can't get my rings on. My right thigh, in particular, aches.

My greatest anxiety is developing a DVT. I must be very high risk and I am so concerned about having to take warfarin for the rest of my life. What an awful thought. I guess I would cope, but the thought appals me at present.

I have noticed that my toes are becoming more numb. I am also getting significant paraesthesia (pins and needles) in both feet. I find it quite difficult to dry them after a shower. I can't feel what I am doing properly!

I'm still getting intermittent 'hot flushes' when I have to take off my hat and jacket, or throw off the duvet to cool off. I have these episodes once or twice most nights, also most evenings and periodically during the day. They are mostly a problem at night.

I have had quite a few migraines in the last week or so. I hadn't had one since I was diagnosed and stopped HRT, but now I have had a run of them. I don't know what's triggered them. It may be due to my level of fatigue – I'm not sure. Fortunately, the headache is never that bad and I'm not sick; I am just getting the rainbow-coloured zigzag lines starting in my left visual field and then moving to the right over about half an hour. I then may or may not get a headache.

The other thing I have noticed recently – which is definitely due to fatigue – is periodic twitching of an eyelid. Again, this is something I haven't had for a long time. The last time it occurred regularly was before I had my glasses changed. It settled as soon as the lenses were adjusted.

I have probably done too much work today, rather than putting my feet up. I spent thirty-five minutes driving to work this morning, even though I was only trying to get to the hospice – two miles away – by road. That certainly won't have helped my legs, but it doesn't explain the swelling of my arms and face! The ward round was constructive, and I managed to do my mosaic. I then spent the afternoon at the rape suite, working for the police, seeing a very vulnerable patient. Trying to do some work and spend time with my daughters is keeping me focused, but I may be expecting too much of myself. I will have to review what I have timetabled for the weekend.

What an up and down day yesterday was! I had set myself a challenge which I really wanted to achieve. I had promised to drive Rachel to Reading to see how well I could manage it.

Learning To Be (the) Patient

Oh what a contrasting day!

We reached Reading in plenty of time. It was misty on the way but the sun was trying to break through. The Chilterns looked beautiful. On the way back I stopped off in Marlow to have a stroll by the Thames. I listened to the mute swans calling to one another – what a misnomer! The Thames was so beautiful glistening in the sunlight. It was so warm. I sat on a bench at the edge of the parish church graveyard looking at the river, wondering for how many hundreds of years Christians had done the same thing. It was good to sit in the church for a while. Apparently, there has been a church at that spot since the tenth or eleventh century. It is a wonderful thought to think that Christians have been praying there for a thousand years.

The trees looked magnificent, especially the cedar of Lebanon covered with cones. The yew trees made me think of my chemotherapy, and I was grateful. It was lovely to watch the long-tailed tits and to hear the goldcrests. There were so many flowers blooming and so many trees coming into leaf.

It was a fantastic walk and Rachel had a great time at her interview.

In the evening I made a major mistake. I was trying to tidy up the lounge and had removed Rachel's coat from the armchair. Nick started to take his shoes off in the lounge, and I found myself saying out loud that I wondered whether the shoes would be left in the middle of the lounge floor. He hit the roof and stormed upstairs. He was fed up of being nagged by me. He was still angry when I went to bed. The treatment's getting to me. I am too tired and preoccupied by the side-effects to be discreet. I am saying things I would normally suppress. I am not as tolerant as I usually am, and I guess he isn't either.

Overnight, I resolved to talk about it first thing in the morning, to try to make him understand that it is not easy to be sensitive all the time, when my mood is affected by dexamethasone, pain, anxiety about side-effects; I also wanted to find out if he wanted me to opt out of the last dose of chemo, as we were struggling to cope. I wasn't trying to be manipulative but I was trying to acknowledge that my treatment was getting more difficult for all of us, and I didn't want us to reach breaking point. We needed time to reflect on ways to keep sane. Perhaps I would be better off entirely on my own.

During the evening Nick was playing chess and Rachel was out at her friend's house. I felt incredibly lonely and down. I was wrong; I do need company. I don't like being left entirely on my own.

Thursday 29 March

I suppose the most constructive time to write up my journal is when my symptoms are at their worst, but when I am exhausted it's hard to get round to it. It's difficult trying to keep this up, but I will keep going as much as I can.

I am really fed up with the fluid retention, my heavy, swollen, fat legs and tight swollen arms. My face seems to get puffier and puffier. I'm not convinced that 40 mg furosemide this morning is helping. When I lie down my legs go down a bit but my face and arms get puffier!

I slept very badly last night. I had dreadful hot flushes and I was terribly restless. I didn't really think I was in pain but I eventually settled after taking ibuprofen. My feet were more comfortable.

I did make some constructive decisions at the hospice this morning, but I wasn't really well enough to work today; I probably shouldn't have worked, and I feel I am doing some embarrassing things without thinking. I am too exhausted mentally and physically to think.

I didn't realise quite how exhausting all this would become. I knew I would get weaker but this is far worse than I had anticipated. Of course, I had continued to arrange to do things, without knowing how much worse I would become during these last few treatments.

On Tuesday evening, the last thing I wanted was to face another treatment. I wanted a break; I wanted to be let off. Surely five treatment cycles would be enough; my body certainly seemed to think so. I thought I had better see how my daughters would react before going any further. I spoke to Marian first, over the phone. She listened very well and was very sympathetic. I felt she would understand if I decided not to have the last dose. I then spoke to Rachel. Her reaction was exactly as I had expected it to be, and what I had maintained from the beginning. I had argued on several occasions that I would complete the course for the sake of my family. If I develop a recurrence without completing the chemo, they would always wonder 'what if', and that wouldn't be fair on them. When I spoke to her, Rachel immediately made it clear she would worry that the treatment hadn't been adequate.

I went to see my GP Andy at the surgery. Their system for cancer patients is very good. He has a special slot at 5.30 p.m. to be allocated on the day to a cancer patient who needs to be seen. We talked about the fluid retention and my worries about the final chemo. He agreed with Rachel that I should have it, but we discussed modifying the dosage of various drugs to try to improve things. It is incredibly useful having my GP also in charge of the day-to-day running of the chemo unit!

I know I have been overdoing things, but when I planned events I thought this would be my 'good week' before my last chemo, not anticipating that the 'good week' wouldn't happen. I wanted to say 'thank you' to everyone in our church home group for their support and the meals they have provided. I invited everyone round to our house for an Indian feast. The local Indian takeaway provided an excellent spread, very reasonably, including free papadoms and pickles. It was delicious and we all enjoyed it. Somehow, I managed to keep going in spite of my symptoms. I am really pleased we managed it, but cleaning and tidying the house, and getting the room ready was quite exhausting. I had also promised to go to the surgery to complete some more paperwork, and there was shopping to do too.

I was very proud of Rachel. She organised a brilliant welcoming activity for the party. As well as getting us to clap rhythms she also got us kneading dough and crushing grapes. First, she made us all go and wash our hands! She is quite a teacher! Whilst we were eating our feast, the bread rose in the airing cupboard, and she then baked it in the oven. At the end of the feast we broke the bread and gave thanks, shared the bread and grape juice as an informal communion. It was a beautiful little activity.

I suppose that after all that, it isn't surprising that I slept badly.

(Amusingly, when I typed that I actually wrote 'spelt badly' rather than 'slept badly'. What a wonderful example of dyslexic typing!)

Friday 30 March

Rachel has gone up to London to spend the day with Marian. They plan to spend the day doing dance classes and learning about a healthy lifestyle. I'm sure they will have a great time. Meanwhile, I am resting in bed still trying to cope with shifting oedema. First thing this morning my ankles didn't look too bad but the tops of my arms were very puffy. I know when they are swollen because, as well as feeling heavy, there is resistance when I hold them against my chest wall. As soon as I sat down at the computer to check my emails this morning, the fluid started to shift, and my ankles started to swell up more, and the skin on the back of my hands is wrinkled again, so no longer as tight! That's why I have taken myself back to bed to try to settle my legs. I have taken furosemide 40 mg this morning and I am passing more urine, but I am also thirsty, so it may not do much good. The problem about going back to bed is that I know the post has come, but I can't just nip downstairs to get it, I will be breathless when I get back upstairs and my pulse will be racing. I noticed this morning that when I have climbed the stairs I am instinctively behaving like the classical emphysematous 'pink puffer', breathing by blowing my breath out slowly through pursed lips to minimise the resistance to the flow. I noticed I was doing this before my last chemo, but it had stopped. Now I am doing it again.

Last night, I had heartburn again, and I am also suffering from oesophageal pain again. This is interesting, as I had noticed that the problem appeared to have resolved, and I was able to sleep on two pillows rather than three. Last night, I had pain in spite of sleeping propped up on three pillows. Why? I'm not sure.

Wow! I have just achieved something! I have confirmed with Nick (senior forensic medical examiner, or police surgeon) that I am not planning to go back to working nights for the police and he is suggesting that we look for another doctor to join the rota. He has reassured me that the others will not mind me only working days. I will need to look at the best way to manage this, but I think I will be able to manage driving backwards and forwards to South Bucks, provided it is only during the day. This means I have definitely reduced my workload when I return to work properly, but I have ensured that my income is reasonable, without police night duty.

Reflection on activities and workload

When I list my symptoms, does that all sound really pathetic?

Am I pushing myself too hard, and then complaining too much? I am still thinking about going up to London tomorrow to go to see a musical with the girls, and I am meant to be covering Aylesbury police station on Sunday. Am I crazy?

As a doctor, I have always driven myself to keep going, treating any minor medical condition affecting me as efficiently as possible, so that I could keep going. Time off was never an option for infections. I still worked in spite of severe pain from a dental abscess, from a breast abscess, and sinusitis, etc. I don't feel guilty about having time off now for my chemotherapy, but I know I am still pushing myself to do as much as I possibly can. Will I look back and think I was an absolute idiot to try to do so many things during my chemotherapy, or will I regret not achieving enough during my extended time off?

At the moment I look back and wonder how I managed to fit in so much into the time I had before I became ill. How did I ever keep going, especially after a night on call for the police?

I said I was fine as long as I managed to have an afternoon nap. Was I really? Did the patients I saw the following morning get a raw deal? Yes, possibly, but I was so used to on-call and sleepless nights when the children were younger, it was all part of my lifestyle.

Of course, I made one lifestyle choice to enable me to continue the night-time work relatively safely, and I'm paying for that now. Four years ago I wasn't coping with the night sweats. I wasn't sleeping well on the nights I wasn't on call. I chose to start HRT and it immediately resolved my sleep problem. I knew the risks and considered myself at low risk of developing breast cancer, so considered it a risk worth taking. I still think it was, and I know I must continue to be objective when I talk to patients about HRT.

Concerning my breast cancer, I do wonder if all the on-call I did and the excessive hours I worked were also contributing factors. Somehow I managed to keep going but my body has suffered. I cannot do it again safely.

Saturday 31 March

I've lost a bit of weight but I am still breathless going up and downstairs. I'm not going to London. My legs would be so uncomfortable after sitting on the train and in the theatre. It's a beautiful day so I may try to go for a short walk on the flat this afternoon, otherwise I will recline on the settee and watch world cup cricket and *Dr Who*! People seem to think that I have been watching a lot of daytime television. It's hasn't been true up until now, but the oedema has forced me to rest more. The easiest thing to do when resting on the settee is to watch cricket. It requires little effort!

April 2007

Tuesday 3 April

Today is blood test day, and outpatient appointment day, before the last chemo tomorrow. I really don't want it, I really don't want to live with these side-effects for another three weeks (at least), but somehow I will keep going.

It's special that it's Holy Week. By Good Friday I will be exhausted. I am also getting a lot of pain in my upper arm muscles. Initially, it was just my left arm, after moving the guinea pig run on Sunday, hammering all the pegs back into the ground after the little girl escaped. At least she is back safely in the run.

Last night we went to see *Amazing Grace*, the film about Wilberforce and the abolition of the slave trade. It was an excellent film, and very moving. What a great Christian message of perseverance in the face of years of opposition, as well as ill health. They also depicted the problems of managing chronic abdominal pain with opium very well, showing Wilberforce's decisions to withdraw 'cold turkey', so he could think clearly during the debate of his abolition bill. His life was depicted warts and all, but the virtuous Christian life shines through.

I wasn't feeling great today but it was good to go into day hospice. Patients and staff were very supportive. Unfortunately, I missed the Easter service in the afternoon, because I had to go to outpatients. My arms are still aching and very uncomfortable. I talked to one patient today whose main complaint is a constant ache in his left arm. My experience certainly helped my understanding of his problem.

My white cell count is fine but if only I were feeling better today. I don't feel ready for the next dose of chemo, but I'm certainly not postponing it. It will be a great relief when it is all over.

Wednesday 4 April

I woke up this morning and realised I had slept quite well, and all the pains in my arms had disappeared. The relief was huge but, of course, it is due to going back on dexamethasone. The relief of muscle pain by steroids, within twenty-four to forty-eight hours of commencing the drug, is used to help diagnose polymyalgia rheumatica, an inflammatory muscle disorder. Is this something else I've got to put up with? Just when I am looking forward to a time without too much medication, and a reduction in the side-effects, I'm suddenly confronted with the possibility that I will develop significant muscle pain and weakness again on stopping dexamethasone – the drug I hate taking – but with the knowledge that restarting it would relieve the pain. Is there a chemotherapy-induced polymyalgia-type syndrome? Is this exactly what people with the disease suffer from? I've had several migraines recently but at least I haven't had tenderness over my temporal arteries, which would make it even more serious.

Stop it Hazel!

I must stop diagnosing myself, and behaving like a neurotic doctor! I am sure that the effect will be transient, and I will cope with it, but it is important to document it, so that I have an accurate record if it does recur.

My mood was better this morning, as well, when I woke up. This, again, is the effect of dexamethasone. I made sure I got to the midweek communion and to the cancer and chemotherapy unit this morning. It was good to have Rachel with me for the last treatment. We both wore our new hats and I sat next to my friend having herceptin, so we had a lovely chat throughout the session. Sadly, one of her friends, who had her surgery at the same time as she did, has a recurrence in her hip. We talked about this, and her long-term management, but naturally, my friend has mixed emotions and doesn't know what to say to her. She feels sad for her friend, but relieved it's not her, but guilty that she feels like that.

After my chemo Rachel and I went to the hospice so I could show her my mosaic. She was very impressed, but I've still got several weeks work to go before it's complete.

Maundy Thursday

I had a very quiet morning, but the weather was so beautiful I decided to go for a walk before my afternoon nap. The sky was blue, the weather incredibly warm, and there was no breeze, so I went to Wilstone reservoir. One of the highlights was seeing three lively bunnies romping in the field, including one black one. It was wonderful to see beautiful brimstone butterflies and small tortoiseshell butterflies enjoying the warmth. Not many water birds around except about twenty herons' nests, and three babies, clearly visible, in one of the nests. It was lovely to hear the chiffchaffs, chaffinches, robins, and wrens singing, and one blackcap. I wonder if the chiffchaffs and blackcaps have flown in from abroad, or whether they have over wintered here. Most of the over wintering ducks have gone, just a few wigeon left, but the terns, sand martins and hobbies don't seem to have arrived yet.

It's a wonderful time of year, with the leaves coming on the trees, and the song birds singing their hearts out. The reservoir banks were covered with celandines, but I couldn't find the lovely cowslips that are usually bloom at this time of year. They must have been disturbed by the renovation work that took place over the winter.

Good Friday

I hadn't expected to be able to get up in time to go to the 10.30 a.m. meditation around the cross this morning, but I did. This was very special. It has also been good to reflect again on the *Seven Last Words of our Saviour from the Cross*, listening to the Haydn string quartet, played by the Lindsays. I found our copy yesterday whilst tidying up. I had completely forgotten we had a copy, and the CD was still in the wrapper. Yesterday was the perfect time to find it!

Spiritual reflection

I felt very weak as I walked down to the school, to the Oaks Community Church service this morning. Jesus had been beaten over the head, and flogged, and dragged from one place to another, all night. No wonder he was exhausted, and couldn't carry his cross. Some of the written words in the meditation reflected on Jesus's weakness, his humanity, his frailty. Walking down the hill, and back up again this morning, I couldn't have carried even one bag of shopping; I was too weak. I am so relieved my chemotherapy is over. I will gradually get my strength back. Jesus suffered for us all, it is good to be reminded of his suffering. My suffering has been trivial in comparison, but I too am coming to the end of that long journey.

Whilst I am writing this, Rachel is practising the prayer from Jewish Life *by Bloch on her cello. Listening to the cello 'crying' in the minor key reminds me of Jesus weeping over Jerusalem, and the women weeping over his death. So amazingly appropriate.*

Good Friday is a special time for reflection, but it has also been another beautifully sunny and warm day. The Independent *this morning had a series of poems for spring. Reading Wordsworth's poem again made me think.*

> I wandered lonely as a cloud
> That floats on high o'er vales and hills,
> When all at once I saw a crowd,
> A host, of golden daffodils;
> Beside the lake, beneath the trees,
> Fluttering and dancing in the breeze.
>
> Continuous as the stars that shine
> And twinkle on the milky way,
> They stretched in never-ending line
> Along the margin of the bay:
> Ten thousand saw I at a glance,
> Tossing their heads in sprightly dance.

The waves beside them danced; but they
Out-did the sparkling waves in glee:
A poet could not but be gay,
In such jocund company:
I gazed – and gazed – but little thought
What wealth the show to me had brought:

For oft, when on my couch I lie
In vacant or in pensive mood,
They flash upon that inward eye
Which is the bliss of solitude;
And then my heart with pleasure fills,
And dances with the daffodils.

Oh how I would love to express my feelings in such a wonderful way. If only I could speak out my feelings of praise and wonder when I go for a walk, and see the beauty of God's creation. If only I could convey the depth of feeling, of awe and wonder. I'm so grateful we have the psalms, music and these poems to share and enjoy. Words that express what I want to say, and music that brings out the feelings that well up inside me, as I look at and remember the wonderful things I saw with Rachel today. I love Wordsworth's last verse; it's so special, as I sit on my couch, remembering the beauty of the day. At least my mind can dance with the flowers, and enjoy the echoes of the skylark, chiffchaffs and wrens ringing in my ears. Yes, my heart does fill with pleasure!

I went again to Wilstone reservoir and we walked all round, up to the canal (undergoing restoration) and back to the hide. We had some wonderful views of great-crested grebes, a skylark was singing in the field, and we heard so many chiffchaffs. We both agreed they should be called chiff-chiffchaffs, as they call out in three-time and not two-time! Where it was warm we saw several peacock butterflies, and there was a whole carpet of violets under the trees. From the hide the snipe seem to have gone, but there were two goldeneyes. I am sure they will be off up north very shortly!

As we drove back there are so many trees covered in blossom. It won't be long before the horse chestnuts are in flower either.

A few lines of A.E. Housman's poem sums up the beauty of the trees in Spring:

> Loveliest of trees, the cherry now
> Is hung with bloom along the bough,
> And stands about the woodland ride
> Wearing white for Eastertide.

One final quote from this morning's paper, a thought by Robert Orben: 'Spring is God's way of saying, "One more time!"'

How do I interpret that? Jesus died to give us another chance; death and resurrection are re-enacted every year in the spring. One more time, God is reminding us, calling us back into relationship with Him.

Easter Saturday – three days post-chemo

Rachel complained I was stressed and irritable this morning, and then went, as arranged, to visit grandma. My energy levels were very low. I managed some ironing in the morning, and then a very slow trip to the shops, via the carwash. I don't know how I managed to dash round the car, checking the tyre pressures in less than two minutes. It wore me out, but it made me realise how foolish I had been. I doubt I have checked the pressures (and they were much lower than they should be) since I became ill. OK, I don't use the car much but that's not the point. I must check the oil!

What other things have been neglected whilst I have been ill? I sat down to read some of my medical papers and journals. My concentration wasn't good, but I realised how medical politics and medicine has moved on. I'm worried I've been left behind. I will need to do some updating before July. There was a philosophical letter in one of the papers about how GPs had concentrated so hard, trying to gain as many quality points as possible – to prove they are providing a quality service, and to gain income – that the relationship, built up over years, between the doctor and the patient (family) has been neglected. That is definitely not true of our practice, and is one of the reasons why we won't be near the top of the pile when the quality points are published. I am glad that patients still come first in our practice, but can we keep it that way?

The trip to Tesco exhausted me. The supermarket trolley kept me upright, but I was walking so slowly. I can't go up and down all the aisles; that would be far too far to walk. By the time I got home for lunch, I just wanted to go to bed. When I woke again, well after 4 p.m., I lay in bed, thinking about the housework that would confront me when I got downstairs – vacuuming, and clearing the clotheshorse, which was occupying a large amount of space in the lounge. The trouble was, I knew that that would involve several trips up and downstairs – could I manage that?

Nick came home from watching football as I finished the work. I wasn't good company. I was happy to quietly watch television, but I had a headache. Why did he decide to create a racket just before we had supper? Wasn't he aware of my body language? Didn't he hear me quietly saying 'shhhh' earlier? This is exactly what happened three weeks ago, on the last Saturday after my chemo, when we went shopping together. He was singing and taking his time in the supermarket when all I wanted to do was go home. I had had enough; he was oblivious. At least I went shopping on my own today, so I was independent, and free to stop when I wanted to.

The sweats started after supper. One minute I was feeling cold and looking for my hat and blanket, the next I was pouring sweat from the back of my neck. My legs were uncomfortable; I felt really poisoned. When I got to bed I was very restless, my hands felt really cold, and then I started sweating again. I lay in bed wondering why on earth I had gone through this final treatment cycle – this final torture. Was the family going to be able to cope with it? Was I going to get better? Hadn't I had enough after the last cycle? When would it all end? What would happen to my weight over the next few days? Would the fluid all come back, and make me really breathless again, and how would I get rid of it? My thoughts were all jumbled; I suppose I kept drifting off to sleep for a few moments, but I had noticed this happened last cycle too. I suppose it's another aspect of the poisoning – incoherent thinking!

Easter Sunday

I made it to church with Marian in the morning, but then had to go back to bed rather than cooking Sunday lunch. Much to my delight, Marian cooked it for us. I managed to muster the energy to move the guinea pig run, but it was really another very hard, rather unpleasant day.

Easter Monday

I got my energy back today! Cleaning, washing, ironing, sorting out and packing to go to Spring Harvest. Moreover, I went with the girls to Thame Country Show, and walked round the stands at the showground for a couple of hours. It was so warm; I was too hot wearing my hat, so I took it off. My hair has grown back sufficiently now for me not to worry too much whether I wear one or not.

Highlights of the day included the South of England hamster show, the local rabbit show, Harris hawks and some owls, and of course the red kites overhead. It was also lovely to hear the skylarks. Oh, how I love the song of the skylark, which always brings back memories of the times we have had in the Shetlands, where there are so many. The skylark is so much part of the disappearing British countryside; it was not a great surprise to me, when it was announced today, that Vaughan-Williams's *Lark Ascending* was voted top of the Classic FM Hall of Fame this year.

Tuesday 10 April

Well, Rachel has gone back to Manchester, and Marian is on the way with us to Spring Harvest. It was wonderful to see the buzzards circling on the way – three circling together, enjoying the thermals. The sun is still shining and it is still ridiculously warm.

Friday 13 April – Day four at Spring Harvest

The weather was not quite as good today, but we spent time on the beach yesterday, and Nick actually swam!

It is so easy to be too busy here to reflect on what is happening. One talk merges into another, and one day into the next. This afternoon it is important to sleep and reflect.

Notes for reflection:
- We have lost our understanding of awe. Everyone has a moment in life which can really be described as awesome – but what?
- Yesterday, I was feeling sorry for myself as I was unable to do all that I would have liked to do. I have reached the end of the first part of my journey – how flexible am I? I need to live with uncertainty, but am I ready and open to what God has prepared for me next? I've got rather comfortable in the dual role of doctor and patient. Am I ready for my next challenge?

Saturday 14 April

Nick and Marian both swam in the sea!

I asked Marian if she had a moment in her life that was truly 'awesome'. I made the comment that I often hear her and Rachel using the term when something special has happened but I meant something much greater than that.

I reminded her of the moment in Wind in the Willows *when Mole and Ratty find the baby otter . It is a profoundly spiritual moment and they are afraid. Or the experience that Peter, James and John had when they saw Jesus transfigured. Something so amazing that, whatever happened to them in the future, they could look back on that moment to strengthen their faith. Had she had that sort of spiritual moment when she was overwhelmed by the greatness, and holiness of God, and his love?*

She said she had had a special experience shortly after joining Kensington Temple.

I reflected that I had had the special moment shortly after I was diagnosed with cancer when I went for a walk along the canal. I experienced the amazing sight of the moon rising and illuminating a solitary bush in such a way that I couldn't keep my eyes off it; it was so beautiful. It was a profoundly spiritual moment. I was so clearly reminded of the story of Moses and the burning bush, and God revealing himself to Moses. I knew the Lord was saying to me my cancer journey would be a long one but he would be with me, watching over me constantly. He didn't promise me a smooth journey but he did promise to be with me throughout.

I have often thought about that moment when I have needed encouragement, and the memory has given me the strength to continue.

I also mentioned one other moment in my life that has stuck in my mind and strengthened my faith. It was when I was a medical student. I was alone standing beside a secluded pond, looking at the water. I felt the Lord telling me to take my glasses off. I am quite short-sighted, and I took my glasses off which meant everything was pretty blurred and indistinct. I then put them back on again and the water and the vegetation came into focus again. I felt that the Lord was saying that the difference between what I saw without my glasses, and what I saw with them on, is the contrast between what the world is like now, and what Heaven will be like. Everything will be so much more beautiful and more sharply focused. Before this revelation I had been moaning that I was fed up with having to wear glasses, after all I was young and wanted to look my best! After this special moment I realised that if I had perfect eyesight I wouldn't have received this revelation.

There have been many other special moments, but these two are experiences that I will never forget and really help to maintain and strengthen my faith.

Sunday 15 April – Last day at Spring Harvest

Whilst Nick was driving us home I pondered whether we had enough fresh ingredients in the fridge to cook an evening meal after all we had had rather mediocre fare for the last few days as half-board guests at Butlins (I hasten to add we enjoyed the breakfasts!). But it would be good to have 'fresh' ingredients. A vegetable omelette came to mind.

I cut my thumb whilst slicing a tomato (only a minor cut!). I wasn't using a chopping board but, as I am accustomed to doing, I was holding the tomato in my right hand and cutting it with my left.

I know I should be more sensible but I have always sliced vegetables like that and always been safe until now. I should have thought that it's been several days since I prepared a meal; the feeling in my fingers and toes isn't as good as it should be; I'm a bit more clumsy than normal. I remembered when I cut myself. I needed to see the blood to convince myself it had happened because I hardly felt it. It didn't hurt.

Now I know how important it is for diabetics to understand foot (and hand) care. Obviously, leprosy is a third-world example. I trust my peripheral neuropathy is transient but theirs isn't. Risk-taking is dangerous. I was stupid. My white cell count may still be low. I washed the cut well but I risked a significant infection.

Monday 16 April

My glasses felt comfortable when I put them on this morning but I'm worried that they won't be for long. Yesterday evening I took 40 mg furosemide and I have taken some this morning. I didn't want to take a diuretic prior to travelling home in the car from Minehead for fairly obvious reasons! I can see why patients take their diuretics intermittently, omitting them if they are going out, especially if they are not in control of 'loo stops' or they don't know the area and where the public toilets are. There is a downside to omitting the medication. Yesterday, I was drinking plenty but didn't even need to go to the loo when we reached home four hours later. My legs had swollen up badly again and by the evening my head was so swollen that my glasses had produced a deep ridge above my ears. This had happened before but this time it was so uncomfortable I had to take them off.

I can't see without my glasses. I wear them all the time, except when I'm asleep. What can I do?

I started to feel sorry for myself again last night. I was frustrated with myself. But then is it so unreasonable to be upset when something fundamental to daily living becomes a problem?

This is the sort of experience I always dread when I get new glasses; when I can never be sure initially whether they are comfortable or not, but if they are tight after a while, at least you have the old pair to change to, until the new are corrected.

I really don't know what to do with this pair today. On the one hand, if I go to the optician and get them adjusted (if that is possible) the situation is only going to be temporary. They will be far too loose in a few days' time, when the swelling subsides. Anyway, it is a bit of a walk to the opticians from the car park; I'm not sure I could make it. On the other hand, today I have to drive to Oxford for my radiotherapy planning appointment. Maybe my prescription sunglasses will be looser. That's a thought, but I don't know, as I haven't worn them for months. Tomorrow I am meant to be working. How can I work if my glasses aren't comfortable?

Anyway, I'm not sure where the sunglasses are.

Spring Harvest was great. Yesterday morning ended on a real 'high'. A proper mountain-top experience, a mood-lifting and faith-building experience like Peter, James and John's experience when they witnessed 'the transfiguration' of Jesus. The trouble is you have to come back down the mountain, and get back to the daily grind, and face up to your problems. For a short time yesterday I was walking well on the flat, keeping up with the crowd; my mood was good, I was really beginning to feel better. But by evening, back home I had to face up to the problems of so much fluid retention.

Good news! I remembered my sunglasses had fallen down under the passenger seat in Nick's car. He had cycled to work so the car was parked in the drive. When I tried them on they are definitely looser and more comfortable. When the swelling goes down they will need adjusting as they will keep slipping down, but they are just right now, and I managed to drive to Oxford and back without incident. The thought that came to me – to try my sunglasses – was definitely inspired!

By lunchtime today I was definitely more relaxed. Spring Harvest has certainly helped! My sense of humour surprised me today. As I was driving past the police station I spotted the notice by the entrance saying 'All visitor parking suspended during construction work'. In the past the notice has just frustrated me, as I like to park by the duck pond at the front of the building when visiting the police station, but this time a picture came straight into my head of my car hanging in mid-air! At least it's not arrests that are being suspended…

My radiotherapy planning appointment was good. The radiographers were very friendly, but competent and professional. It was good to have a longer chat with Amanda, my consultant. She spotted my nails, with four clear Beau's lines (ridges) across them. A medical student had a good look too. I must try to photograph them. It is amusing to reflect that my father wrote the definitive text book *The Nails in Disease* with excellent photos. If he were still alive he would be very impressed by his daughter's nails.

I have never been into a radiotherapy treatment room before. I wondered if it would be 'scary' but, in fact the room was large and airy, and I was put at ease, even though lying on the treatment couch with my arms above my head for about half an hour was rather uncomfortable.

I was told I was a very good patient and the planning went very smoothly. I now have four tiny tattooed markers on my chest wall. My first tattoos at the age of fifty!

Amanda asked me to sign the consent form pointing out that the aim of radiotherapy is to avoid local recurrence. I agreed wholeheartedly, saying that local recurrence was my worst nightmare. I then told her that, in fact, I had had a nightmare about that very thing; we talked about the patient, who we both remembered very well, whose disease had triggered my dream. It was suddenly good to talk as colleagues with a shared experience, both still struggling to come to terms with what had happened to that patient, but also reinforcing the importance for me of having all the appropriate treatment.

It was also good to laugh during our discussion. She asked me to sign a form confirming that I am not pregnant! I was highly amused pointing out that I had a mirena coil, I hadn't had a period for many months, I had been on HRT for menopausal symptoms and I was certainly getting hot flushes now. Also, I had just completed a course of chemotherapy… and as I signed the form I added as an afterthought: and, of course my husband had a vasectomy twenty years ago. No, I am not pregnant!

Tuesday 17 April

I had my hair cut and styled in day hospice today. It's nice and neat and tidy now but it will be a while before I get a fringe again! I wish it wasn't quite so grey! My eyebrows are still half-missing.

I have been working at the hospice this morning and being creative in day hospice this afternoon as well as covering the police station. I coped quite well with the police work today. I saw two people arrested on suspicion of murder. They both seemed polite, nice young men. I really don't know, but neither of them was behaving as if they had anything to worry about.

In spite of having very uncomfortably swollen legs, I am very reassured that I managed to cope with the workload and enjoyed it. This is an important turning point as I am beginning to realise that I do enjoy my work, gain a great deal from it, and flourish through contact with people and hearing their stories.

One of the patients at the hospice today was a challenge for me. The patient was young and had been diagnosed with cancer at the same time as me and had surgery around about the same time, but her cancer had recurred. My colleagues were concerned that I might not cope. I didn't feel that would be a problem but I was concerned the patient might not cope with seeing me. It is quite obvious to patients that I have just had chemotherapy, especially as I have stopped wearing a hat now and my face is puffy with little in the way of eyelashes or eyebrows.

I'm not sure the patient who was wearing a hat noticed my appearance. But I noticed how black the patient's mood was. Yes, if I had gone through surgery and all these cycles of treatment and then discovered I already had widespread disease my mood would be low; it's totally understandable.

Wednesday 18 April
<u>Reflection on my journey</u>

It was good to reflect on the patient's story yesterday. I am grateful my journey is continuing; I still have work to do. This week has been a turning point. I am beginning to enjoy and be encouraged by my work again. It is important to me. I love my work, as long as I don't become overwhelmed by it.

One lesson I need to learn from my extended sick leave is that my work is a special and very significant part of my life, but I must have time to reflect and learn from my patients. Over the last few years the patients that I have written about in my casebooks and my dissertation are the ones from whom I have gained the most. Exploring and thinking about their family dynamics, or exploring the ethical issues in their management, has been so rewarding and constructive for the management of other patients – not least me as the patient!

Conclusion: I must keep my workload under control both for my family's sake and to maintain the quality of work. The patients will benefit when I have time to reflect and I need to ensure that this doesn't get pushed aside. Tiredness will do this.

New symptoms

My arms are starting to ache around the elbows again. I really didn't want this to happen again. This was what happened last cycle and only disappeared when I started back on dexamethasone. I am not going back on dexamethasone. I have finished my chemo, so I don't know how to manage it. This could be the start of a rather rough part of my journey.

Friday 20 April

It is not easy to keep this journal up to date. There are so many other things to do as well. Yesterday was an extremely busy day. I worked hard at the hospice in the morning, but it was rewarding. I then popped into town to see my old colleagues from the family planning clinic before going to my theology tutorial. After a short sleep, I drove to Amersham for a meal with the other police surgeons. Last night my arms ached and I certainly need a quiet day today.

Sunday 22 April

My energy levels are picking up and I am beginning to feel better. I worked hard in the garden yesterday after a quieter day on Friday. I wasn't very careful pruning the bushes. I was wearing thick gloves to protect my hands to above the wrists but it was so warm I had only a short sleeved top on. At lunchtime I noticed I had been scratched on my right forearm just above the gloves. This, of course, is very careless as this is the arm with compromised lymphatic drainage.

It could be even more of a problem after my radiotherapy, so I must learn a lesson from this. I must keep my arms covered when I am gardening, even when the weather is hot.

Monday 23 April

It was raining this morning, the first rain I have seen for some weeks. Three thoughts went through my mind:
1. The grass needs the rain to grow to keep the guinea pigs happy.
2. My planned walk would be replaced by doing the housework.
3. If the swifts, swallows and martins have arrived they will be flying low over the reservoirs, so I could go and look without going for a walk!

It was good to dust, polish and vacuum downstairs. It's made the house smell nice but it highlighted a few problems as well. I knelt down to look in the cupboard under the stairs and I realised I couldn't get up again, and there was nothing to lean on to push myself up with my arms. I told myself I was being stupid, but then crawled on hands and knees to the stairs, and managed to get upright by 'crawling' up the first two steps. I forget how weak my thigh muscles are until something like that happens. I push up with my arms to get out of a chair but forget that I shouldn't need to do that!

After the cleaning I realised I needed a treat. I could go and have a look at the reservoirs. I parked at Wilstone and climbed the steps. I needed three pauses on the way up to get to the top, but I could hear the swifts as soon as I opened the car door. There were possibly a hundred swifts circling and screeching overhead. It was a wonderful sound. A sound telling me that summer is almost here.

A very kind gentleman advised me to drive on to Startops reservoir at Marsworth to see martins and terns. I had been surprised not to see any common terns at Wilstone.

There were plenty of terns at Marsworth. This was a real treat. I love watching them swooping down over the water to drink, and their call reminds me of the sea and the Shetland Islands. OK, the common terns breed here on the freshwater reservoirs as far away from the sea as they can be; it's the arctic tern that breeds on the shingle in the Shetlands, but it is still a wonderful sound and sight, and I can dream!

There were many sand martins flying over the reservoir too, and the occasional swallow. I know 'one swallow doesn't make a summer', as Aristotle wrote, but it is coming, and it's going to be hot again next weekend.

Tuesday 24 April

What a horrible day! Why aren't I beginning to feel better?

My body is still so swollen with fluid. How much longer am I going to have to take furosemide? I want to cry; I know my mood is depressed. I thought I would be starting to pick up by now.

I slept badly. I just couldn't get comfortable when I woke up during the night. My arms were aching so much; I didn't know where to put them. I really didn't want to get up and go to work. Yesterday, I had got up really slowly. It was 11 a.m. before I had a shower; today I had to be at the hospice around 8.30 a.m.

Was I really well enough to work? At least I have permission to use one of the two parking places right outside the hospice front door, to avoid walking any distance, but I had to do a lot of walking up and down the corridor today, and I struggled. Perhaps I should have phoned in sick, but I hate letting people down at the last minute.

My low mood didn't help. I was so sure I would be feeling better by now. I was exhausted by the time I got home. It was about 2.30 p.m. and I needed a rest. I went to bed and woke up five minutes before Nick came home at 5.45 p.m.

Not a good day. I need a glass (or two) of wine and a hug, but Nick's playing chess!

Spiritual reflection

Spring Harvest was good. Sometimes it takes time for a message to sink in. The celebration on the last morning was probably the best and the talk most meaningful.

Mark Madavan was giving the talk. I noticed that he was talking without notes, and Sheila, our friend from church, had spotted him walking around the site with a white stick, earlier in the week. This puzzled me as he started his talk with some slides of elephants, and said he had been recently watching them in South Africa. I eventually realised he must have 'tunnel vision'.

He then started to talk about a journey he had taken some years ago that had involved driving along a good tarmac road for some miles, but then it changed to a rough track. As it was along the side of a mountain, this was quite dangerous. Eventually, the road became smooth, and safe again but not for long! The route kept changing from rough to smooth and they had children in the back. It took hours. He likened that journey to our Christian journey. God promises to be with us but not that it will always be easy. We have to take the rough with the smooth.

He then explained that when he was younger he was told he was suffering from 'night blindness', but it was only later that the full significance of the symptom was explained to him. He was told that he had retinitis pigmentosa. This causes tunnel vision, and he would slowly go blind and there was no cure. That day everything changed, but nothing changed. His vision was no different after he was told than before, but his whole life had changed; he knew he would go blind. There would be rough times ahead.

It was so good to hear a Christian speaker talking so openly about disability. He was being so honest.

It was also good to hear him talking about his 'journey'. These notes are the journal of my journey, a journey that I recognised as I stood by the canal after sunset as the moon was rising. I knew the Lord was speaking to me. He promised that although the journey would be long he would be with me. But, like Mark said, there would be rough times and smooth times; it wouldn't all be easy. Today, it was important to remind myself of that. I have been having a particularly bumpy ride over the last few weeks and I suppose I was hoping, and praying, that the road would have become smooth again by now. I know it will soon, but I must pray for patience.

That was a very constructive reflection, but I'm going to have a glass of wine now.

Wednesday 25 April

I think I was expecting too much too soon. I am still so weak and swollen. It's now three weeks since my last dose of chemo. Today I would have been due my next dose.

I needed some encouragement. I realised that I could at least be positive, thinking about all the symptoms I won't have to endure again.

I noticed my concentration was improving during the communion service this morning, and my thinking won't become muddled again, like it did following each dose, now I've finished my chemo.

I won't have to endure constipation over the next few days, or nausea.

My taste buds won't be affected. I won't find coffee horrible, and I will be able to enjoy red wine.

My sleep pattern is still a problem, but it won't be disturbed again by the dexamethasone.

I am still breathless and swollen, but it is improving and I'm off the medication that will make it worse.

No more awful mood swings. My mood may be a little low but without having to take dexamethasone my mood won't go very high and then very low. It will stabilise and return to normal.

My heartburn should slowly resolve.

My hair will grow back evenly and my nails will start to grow normally again.

I wonder what will happen to the sweats. Hopefully, the dreadful evening sweats were worse because of the dexamethasone and will settle down.

Over the next few days I shouldn't feel agitated and restless in the evening.

I shouldn't need to sleep most of the time. At least my energy levels should improve.

I don't need to worry about picking up infections from salad and fruit, etc because my white cell count should be fine.

I slept for a short time this afternoon and then went to Wilstone and Startops reservoirs again. I saw about seventeen rabbits including two black ones, quite a few swallows and swifts and plenty of terns on both reservoirs. The weather was beautiful so the swifts were very high. Just as I was about to leave Wilstone I spotted what I had gone to see – a hobby chasing the swallows and then one flying over the reed bed. I had been looking out for them, but had thought they might not have arrived yet as they are said to follow the swallows' migration, and I had only seen one or two swallows until today. One swallow doesn't make a summer, but seeing the hobbies suggests summers coming!

Friday 27 April

Today I ran upstairs and then realised what I had done! I can't remember the last time I ran upstairs. I did it again and then showed Nick when he got home. I had to tell Rachel as well when she phoned; it was such fantastic news. I desperately needed some encouragement and got it!

Saturday 28 April

I went up to London today to the history of medicine lecture. My ankles were already swollen after the train journey and my right leg became particularly uncomfortable during the lecture, but the trip was worth it!

After lunch I met Marian in Regent's Park. It was warm and sunny, and after a rest lying on the lawn covered in daisies, we booked an hour on a pedalo. I managed to get on and off of it! I managed to peddle for an hour and then walk around the park, and to and from the restaurant for tea. We had a great time manoeuvring the boat close to the coots' nests. We saw lots of tiny baby coots, plus two beautiful baby great-crested grebes, one riding on the back of the adult. The babies have lovely black and white stripy heads. It was great to have my camera with me.

It was great to see Marian again and tell her, too, that I had run upstairs!

Sunday 29 April

We had lunch at church today. People said I was looking better. People have been saying that for a while. This time I could actually agree with them. I was also complimented on my hair!

Monday 30 April

My radiotherapy started today. I was very glad that Shirley drove me over to Oxford. It was good to have support and my arms are aching too much to cope with driving; this as well as keeping my arms above my head – and completely still – whilst I have the therapy. It was quite uneventful, but I did think I would have liked to leap off the table whilst the final treatment was going on, but realised it would have been disastrous. The poor radiographers

– I wonder how they cope if that happens. Maybe I will ask them before I complete my thirteen trips!

The trip to Oxford and back is so time-consuming. I don't think I will have time to get to the surgery this week, as I am busy at the hospice on Tuesday and Thursday and radiotherapy is Monday, Wednesday and Friday. That is a busy schedule!

May 2007

Tuesday 1 May

I walked to the hospice this morning (and back). This was a great achievement. I even got there in time.

I nearly completed my mosaic in day hospice today, during the afternoon, but ran out of time. Instead, I will complete it next week on my birthday! That will be a very special birthday treat before I have to go for radiotherapy.

Wednesday 2 May

Body image is a major problem. I am really concerned about this. How do I handle this and go to work? I was told that I could not use deodorant or perfumed soap, etc on the area having radiotherapy, but perspiration has always been a problem. It was OK for the first day or so but it is very warm today and I feel smelly. I keep washing and using baby powder but I have to work tomorrow. How can I possibly talk to patients and colleagues at the hospice smelling of body odour?

I was worried that my skin would become too sore to wear my prosthesis but at the moment that is not an issue. I had discussed the fact that I might not be able to work under those circumstances. I know that some ladies live and work without wearing a prosthesis, but I would be far too embarrassed to do that. I would feel self-conscious but also feel that it would be far to distracting for patients (or colleagues). They too would feel embarrassed. I know my hair is very short but that's something that is quite acceptable to talk and laugh about; a missing boob is rather different! On the other hand, yesterday a breast cancer patient at the hospice, who had just been admitted, looked at me and immediately asked me if I had just had chemo. In front of others she then asked me how many doses of radiotherapy I was having. When I said 'thirteen' she said, 'Oh you are a breast, like me!' The other patient then asked me if I had had a mastectomy, so I confirmed this. The first lady, loudly and completely unselfconsciously, announced to the ward, by pushing her left breast up and down, that that one was her prosthesis and then asked me on which side was my prosthesis!

As normal, I had been sitting down during the entire conversation. She then noticed the stethoscope in my hand and said she hadn't realised I was 'official'; she thought my visit had been social. I explained that chatting to the patients was important.

Thursday 3 May

Driving to work this morning I was still anxious about body odour. In fact, I chose not to walk as I didn't want to be sweaty on arrival, but worrying is only making it worse.

Fortunately, the radiographers said it would be OK to use baby wipes and powder so I tried this morning. It was quite constructive, as it was simple and discreet. At the end of the morning I asked Pat from day hospice confidentially if I was smelly. I chose her because I knew she would be honest and wouldn't be embarrassed. She gave me a hug and said 'no'. This was a real relief.

I have been told the situation should improve as the radiotherapy will destroy the sweat glands anyway. I hope so!

I've started doing exercises for lymphoedema. It is hard to know how much of the swelling of my right arm is oedema that will resolve naturally as my legs and left arm settle down, and how much is due to disturbed lymph drainage. I am sure it is wise to start the exercises, anyway. However, my right upper arm is aching badly. I will need to take ibuprofen before my radiotherapy tomorrow. I hope I sleep tonight. I will need ibuprofen to get off to sleep and paracetamol when I wake in the night to get back to sleep. I am still getting major hot flushes, particularly between three and four in the morning. At least I don't have to get up early tomorrow morning.

Friday 4 May

Nick took me over to the Churchill Hospital in Oxford today. He took the afternoon off. As we were due to go to Northampton for our church weekend away, it was obvious what to do – travel from Aylesbury to Northampton via Oxford, but it worked! We even had some time to spare. We visited a beautiful little nature reserve close to the hospital. I had no idea it was there. It used to belong to C.S. Lewis. I could see why such a lovely, peaceful, secluded wood and pond had inspired the great author. As we wandered slowly up the slope I photographed the bluebells in full bloom. We watched the baby coots on the pond and stared down at hundreds of tadpoles in the shallows. It was wonderful to stand and stare, and reflect. I half expected 'Mr Beaver' to come out form behind a tree!

I must tell the girls about this moment – they will be so jealous – they love the Narnia stories.

Sunday 6 May

A weekend away with the church with excellent food and an amusing speaker but I didn't find it easy. The talks were all on 'healing'. I find the subject of healing quite difficult at times, especially when the speaker seemed to claim the medical profession isn't interested in determining the 'root cause' of illness. What do I spend my time doing? Don't I also have a calling to heal? Isn't one of the most satisfying aspects of my job seeing patients who have been struggling with depression or bereavement beginning to flourish again?

I am very grateful that several church members did come up to me to check I was coping, showing that they understood I might be struggling.

There was one really special moment though during the service this morning. My disabled friend Chris prayed beautifully. He recited psalm 139: 13–14.

'For you created my inmost being;
you knit me together in my mother's womb.
I praise you because I am fearfully and wonderfully made.'
(New international version)

He was so sincere. In spite of his disabilities there was no bitterness; just thanks and praise.

Monday 7 May

A wet bank holiday Monday, and my mood is quite low and I am needing a lot of sleep. Tomorrow is my birthday and I'm working and going to radiotherapy.

My arms were aching a great deal this morning. They are still so weak I even struggle to carry my handbag. At least my skin is not sore after three doses of radiotherapy. My anxiety about body odour is resolving. The baby wipes seem to control the problem reasonably well.

Tuesday 8 May

My birthday!

I had to get up really early this morning to go to the sorting office to collect my 'perishable' parcel that the post office had tried to deliver on Saturday. As Monday was a bank holiday there was no way I could collect the item until today. I was very concerned that my perishable present had been sitting in a box in the sorting office for three days and 'in the post' for four. When I was handed it I realised the contents were fresh flowers, as I had feared.

They are still alive! – beautiful orchids in their own little pots of water to keep them healthy. The two pieces of fern, not in pots, were wilting and appeared beyond resuscitation but in fact revived as soon as they were placed in water. What a joy, and sent from my friends at the surgery. How could I have told them they had died in transit? On the outside of the box there had been a message to the delivery man saying the contents were cut flowers, asking him to leave them with a neighbour if there was no answer as it was a

Saturday delivery, but never mind. I am sure I will be able to use this incident in a talk sometime!

Radiotherapy on my birthday – what a treat! At least we bought tiger prawns and plenty of fruit yesterday, so we can have green Thai curry and fruit salad for birthday tea!

I finished my mosaic in day hospice today and received some beautiful flowers from everyone.

Wednesday 9 May

I went into the surgery today and was overwhelmed by the number of presents I received. I am aware that my mood is quite low at home, on my own, but it picked up amazingly whilst chatting to my colleagues (and friends). Along with all the birthday cards and presents was one letter that really touched me. It was from a young Christian mother who is not ashamed to admit she has dyslexia. She had just heard about my illness and it would have required a significant effort to write to me. She said 'you saw me at surgery last year I think in May, where you helped me so much just listening to me…. I just wanted to let you know I felt God sent me to see you at that time…' I was amazed that that came just after my weekend away. I listened to her problems and remember highlighting the root cause of her problems. It was so therapeutic to receive such a lovely letter emphasising the healing nature of listening. The speaker at the weekend had made some unpleasant generalisations about doctors just dishing out pills and not addressing the root cause of the illness. It hurt me. It was good to have written evidence so quickly that I do help to bring healing.

Thursday 10 May

I like teaching!

I really enjoyed teaching the new junior doctor at the hospice this morning. It was very rewarding. It is so much better taking the opportunity to teach on a subject that comes up naturally, while discussing a patient, rather than just doing a more formal 'teaching session'.

Teaching junior doctors may not pay well but it's so important for the next generation of doctors. After all, it would be nice if the doctors who may look after me when I'm dying know at least as much palliative care as I do!

Friday 11 May

How much longer do I need to keep doing this journal? How much longer will this journey last? Does it end when I complete my radiotherapy? Will all the side-effects be over by then? I still have to start on hormone manipulation treatment after I complete radiotherapy and that is for the next five years. The hot flushes are bad enough already. How much worse will my night's sleep become? How on earth will I cope with more hot flushes and trying to get back to a fuller work schedule? I know I shouldn't be, but I am getting anxious about that.

David, our hospice chaplain, talked about three stages of healing this week. What has already been healed, what is being healed and what will be healed. What has already happened, what continues to happen in life and the full healing after death in eternity. I had been telling him that I was struggling from repeatedly being asked the question 'when are you I going to know whether the treatment and prayer has worked?' There is an assumption that I will be scanned or have blood tests to assess my progress, like the PSA (prostate-specific antigen) test for prostate cancer, which is checked regularly to monitor the disease. I keep explaining that I will only be scanned (apart from scanning the left breast) if I develop symptoms, and I will only ever know that the treatment hasn't worked, *and this is if I develop a recurrence! I have tried to come to terms with this uncertainty but it is hard explaining it to others over and over again. They always seem so surprised and disappointed. I feel as if I am letting them down. I'm afraid that if they were looking for signs of a miracle there is nothing to see.*

Saturday 12 May

I went to my mother's yesterday. I travelled to Beckenham by train. In spite of four different trains plus the tube my ankles didn't swell much. This is beginning to improve. However, I was really struggling to move when I got up from sitting for a while, and I still find it difficult to put on or take off a jacket. I seem so weak. My weakness was brought home to me when I couldn't remove the top from a bottle of bitter lemon. I handed it to my mother with marked osteoarthritis of her hands, and she removed it without any difficulty! I hadn't taken ibuprofen for a couple of days (my muscle pain was less and indigestion worse) but I was so uncomfortable overnight. I was coughing, needing four pillows, and had pain at the top of my leg when lying on my side, and I could hardly walk on getting up this morning, so I decided to take ibuprofen this morning. I was on call for Aylesbury police station and was woken up at 8 a.m. It took me an hour to really get moving this morning, but during the morning whilst in custody I realised that I was moving much better. I think this was due to the ibuprofen. I wonder for how much longer I will have to take it?

I was busy and undertook my first Mental Health Act assessment since October last year. I realised how much I was enjoying myself. I certainly want to start doing assessments again on a more regular basis, but I also like the challenge of talking to the prisoners. Earlier in the week, I had been considering giving up the custody work altogether; I have considerable experience and expertise, but I'm out of practice. I don't want to stop it altogether.

Sunday 13 May

I realised in church this morning that I am thinking much more positively about 'living' again, about getting back to work, being more active and participating in life again.

I had a constructive discussion over coffee after the service with Elaine as well. She is due to have her planning appointment for her radiotherapy tomorrow. I should see her there. I gave her the advice that I had been given to moisturise the skin that will be irradiated with aqueous cream twice a day from now on, rather than starting when she starts her radiotherapy. I told her that my skin was coping well with the radiotherapy. Whether it is due to the cream I started six weeks ago or not, I don't know, but it certainly hasn't done any harm. I will certainly recommend it to my patients.

We talked about the 'ban' on the use of deodorants. I advised her to use plenty of Johnson's baby powder and baby wipes as necessary. I said this was probably best and appeared to work. She agreed I didn't smell!

I am beginning to plan and look forward to our holiday in Devon in the middle of June. If my skin is healthy I would like to exercise in the pool as much as possible to try to strengthen my arms. It will be great to go for walks as well. I've also just booked flights to my favourite holiday destination, one of the most beautiful places on earth, for the last week in June. I'm going to go to Fetlar in the Shetlands for a week. I love the solitude, but I won't feel alone. It's always so noisy there with the song of the skylarks and the cry of the curlews, snipe and the arctic terns. It will be fantastic to see the skuas again and the comical puffins. I hope I will hear the plaintive call of the 'rain goose' or red-throated diver again and see the sweet little red-necked phalarope again.

It will be lovely to go and see the nuns on the island to thank them for their prayers. It will be so special to stay with Peter and Janet again. It should be a great time of reflection and healing. Perhaps that will be the right time to finish my journal, the end of this part of my journey.

Tuesday 15 May

I was incredibly excited this morning. I was like a little child waiting for her birthday presents! After 'handover' at the hospice I ran as fast as I could (a very slow jog) down to day hospice but Margaret hadn't arrived. The healthcare assistants promised to let me know when she arrived. An hour later I was given the message. I couldn't wait; I went straight back and there, on the craft table displayed for all to see, was my mosaic! I had completed the tiling of the crane surrounded by lotus flowers last week, but Margaret had taken it home to be grouted. She used brown grout and it looks fantastic!

Reflection on benefits of day hospice

Within weeks of my diagnosis I had asked Margaret if I could construct a mosaic. She gave me an unfinished picture of two doves to practise on and I was hooked! I chose the picture of a crane from a photo in a book of ancient and modern mosaics and Margaret drew the bird outline on a board. That was the Tuesday that I discovered I needed a mastectomy, so I didn't start work on the mosaic until after I had had my surgery. I started doing the outline of the crane in December and it is now finished. It has been so much part of my cancer journey. Making it has been so therapeutic. Four weeks ago, I was feeling very low and tired because I had really hoped I would be feeling better three weeks after my last dose of chemo. I had found it hard in the morning working with the in-patients at the hospice, but going down to day hospice and spending an hour working on the mosaic settled me. I wasn't at all sociable; I just wanted to concentrate on the one thing. Patients and staff recognised my need and respected that. I apologised later for being 'stroppy' but they said they realised I was tired and a bit low. It is such a therapeutic environment. You can 'be yourself' and explore your feelings in the way that is most appropriate for you. It's great; I must be in a unique situation. I can switch from doctor in the morning to patient in the afternoon without anyone questioning my role!

I am now deciding how to display the mosaic and planning my next. When I first started making the crane I resolved to produce two mosaics so that each of my daughters could have one if the cancer progresses, in memory of mum's journey.

Wednesday 16 May

I feel very swollen again today. My rings are too tight, the top of my arms are swollen and so are my feet. I stood on the scales and I had gained four pounds in twenty-four hours. I had tried to reduce my diuretics from 40 mg furosemide daily to 40 mg and 20 mg on alternate days but I need to go back to 40 mg daily. I wonder how long I will need to be on that dose.

Despite my increase in weight I am very pleased with myself, because last night I completed my first-ever theology essay. I have thoroughly enjoyed writing it and thinking logically. It was such fun planning it and composing sentences in my head whilst doing the housework, keeping my brain active! I hope it is good enough. It has been good to do some academic work again. It is something I need to continue in the future.

Today I had my seventh dose of radiotherapy. This is the first time my skin has felt as if it has been sunburnt. It looks quite pink. I hope it doesn't start blistering. At least I have two free days before my next trip to Oxford. Because I am being treated on Saturday, it also means I will have a further two-day break before the next one. I hope that will give my skin time to recover.

I have been so fortunate! Members of my church are taking me over to Oxford and back for my radiotherapy. I couldn't possibly be driving each day it would be far too tiring. I am so grateful to them all for giving up their time like this.

Sunday 20 May

It's getting harder to keep up this journal. This week I worked at the hospice Tuesday and Thursday mornings and had a nap during the afternoon; oh, and I had a theology tutorial on Thursday afternoon, before I went to sleep. Monday, Wednesday and Saturday I had my trips to Oxford for radiotherapy, which are three-hour round trips. My only day off was Friday but I went into the surgery in the morning, and after a sleep in the afternoon, I went up to London.

Radiotherapy plus hospice work feels like a full-time job at present and I need so much sleep!

The trip to London was my birthday present from Marian. She had bought tickets for us to see *The Drowsy Chaperone* at the Novello Theatre. It was hilarious! We dined at Planet Hollywood. They had a meal deal, and much to my delight it was very pleasant and the food was good. We had plenty of time to chat before the performance.

My biggest problem still is ankle swelling. When sitting at a desk looking at the PC I'm uncomfortable even after fifteen minutes. This journal would not have happened if I hadn't bought a laptop at Christmas!

London trips have to be planned so carefully in advance. Sitting on the train for fifty minutes on the way, sitting in a restaurant, sitting in the theatre; leg room is so important. I really struggled on the train going home. My ankles ached so much. I eventually managed to put my feet up on the seat in front for the last ten minutes of the journey. I did slip my shoes off first, unlike the gentleman opposite.

The good news, though, was that the show was on at the same theatre as *The Tempest* had been. Marian took me there with her friends just before Easter, just before my last chemo. On Friday we walked all the way from Piccadilly down the Strand to the theatre; before Easter I met her at Covent Garden, the nearest tube to the theatre, and was exhausted by the short walk. We were in the stalls on that occasion. I would never have made it up to the balcony. I made it without much difficulty on Friday. My exercise tolerance is improving!

You ought to see me when I get up first thing in the morning, though. I am so stiff I can hardly move. I have to go downstairs one step at a time leaning on to the banister, every step hurts. Slowly, over the next hour, I loosen up and I can move more freely.

Today we had a special church service and farewell lunch for our vicar and his wife, Laurence and Cathie. I shall really miss them. It was a great last service.

This afternoon I had my annual trip to Shaftsbury House to take the afternoon service. It was good to reflect on my journey and the story of the Good Samaritan, thinking about 'who is my neighbour'.

After the service I needed to get home to get my bra off, and, of course, my right breast prosthesis, and have my afternoon sleep. My skin is coping pretty well with the radiotherapy, but it gets quite sore around the chest wall where my bra causes pressure. The skin is pink and during the last two doses of therapy I have noticed the whole area feels hot. There is also a sore area over my back which I can't see. I am trying to follow all the instructions. I am washing the area with aqueous cream and applying it after the shower, and not using deodorant. I am looking forward to being able to use deodorant again. It is hard work trying to keep fresh as the weather is warming up. I do get sweaty; baby wipes help but it isn't very nice.

My prayer is that my skin remains intact. I really want to be able to swim in the leisure pool at the hotel we are staying at in Devon next month. It will be such good physiotherapy for me, in relative privacy. I need to experiment with the sponge prosthesis, for swimming, without feeling embarrassed. At present this is really important to me.

Tuesday 22 May

I had a relatively quiet day yesterday because the car was being serviced, however I walked the mile or so back from the garage without getting breathless and then cleaned the kitchen and the bathroom, all by 11 a.m. This is real progress. I have only been cleaning one room at a time over the last few months.

Norman, one of the clergy, took me to Oxford for my radiotherapy today. He asked if it would be OK if his wife Yvonne came too, so she could visit an old friend. As a lad Norman lived in that area and had some wonderful stories to tell; I was so amused. We dropped Yvonne off opposite an old bakery, now a workshop, but not just any old workshop – it was the specialist string instrument restorer's workshop where we had bought Rachel's latest cello. I recalled that the building still retained some of the features of the old bakery. Norman recalled the days when he was a lad when, at the weekend, he used to help deliver bread. The name of one of the customers to whom he delivered bread was C.S. Lewis. But as he said, at the time he had no idea who he was! However, I told him I was sure the story could be used in a sermon, somehow… sharing bread?

I was so amused by this 'coincidence'. I had to tell both daughters about the old bakery and about Norman delivering bread to C.S. Lewis. They loved the story. Well, they still love the Narnia stories. Marian even acted in one last summer.

My right chest wall is getting more painful and I am spending more time at home without my bra on. This means I can't wear my prosthesis. I hope no one comes to the door! I may not be able to work next week, but we will see. I will try the sponge prosthesis rather than the silicon prosthesis but I have to be more careful when wearing the lightweight sponge. When I raise my arm it doesn't move so naturally and when I lower it again the sponge prosthesis tends to stay high on the chest wall, and I become lopsided.

As I am starting to feel better mentally and physically (apart from the pain from radiotherapy) I thought I would start to look back over my journal entries for the beginning of the year. My style has changed and I needed to improve the sentence structure. I thought it would be easy but I suddenly came across my entry when I was in total despair (15 January), when the symptoms were so awful after chemotherapy. It was a shock to read it. I had to stop. I know I have been through a lot, but things are beginning to improve now. Did I really feel like that? How are others going to feel if they read that? I stood up in church and told people that I had felt like that, and wrote to others. What on earth must they have felt like? It must have been really shocking. What must it have been like for my family? I really was desperate. They must have been so, so worried. It's strange, I can tell the story and recount my feelings, but, I suppose, I distance myself from it, recounting it like the case history of one of my patients; seeing the thoughts that I had written down at the time was different. They took me by surprise. Of course I hadn't forgotten the experience but I suppose I had blanked out some of the awful details and they have again hit me very hard.

Wednesday 23 May

I've been looking at last year's appointments diary. I didn't keep a journal of my experiences until I became ill, apart from a list and comments about birds and other animals I had seen, but of course I had an appointments diary. It was really strange looking at it again.

All those fixed entries, important events that I had to attend, my on-call nights for Thames Valley police and, most importantly, our trip to China in October. When I wrote those entries in the diary it never crossed my mind that they wouldn't happen, or we wouldn't be going to China. It brought home the enormity of the event that had changed our lives. My cancer had altered the lives of so many people. Now, the fact we didn't go to China seems trivial, but at the time it was a huge loss for my husband who had really been looking forward to it. It had been his choice of destination, his big trip.

Just before I was diagnosed Marian had made a decision not to take a six-month touring acting job, but instead to stay in London. In the light of subsequent events this was a decision for which I will always be grateful. Her support has been invaluable. However, I am sure my illness has also affected subsequent decisions as well. My illness also made sure my sister and brother-in-law in San Diego visited the UK in March this year, even though they had also done the trip last summer.

Thursday 24 May

I've been waking up terribly early lately, and today is no exception. I decided today to get up and come downstairs just after 6 a.m. Rather than lying in bed attempting to doze and thinking about what to write, I would get up and actually write something!

Yesterday was a gorgeous day; the weather was wonderful. I went for a walk in the afternoon, initially to College Lake and then on to Wilstone reservoir. As usual it was the terns that mesmerised me, hovering over the water and then swooping down to brush the surface or diving down to catch a fish.

I had a lovely chat with Sandra from next door. They have been on a wonderful cruise. I did have a short nap before cooking tea but I am really pleased with my progress. I coped well with a lot of activities yesterday; after all we then went out to our small midweek church group meeting at Shirley's in the evening. It was beautiful out in the country with the windows open. It was so noisy! The chaffinches, blackbirds, goldcrests and robins, to name a few of the thirteen or so species of birds I could hear singing in the trees outside. There was even a tawny owl later in the evening.

I'm trying to keep cool. With the temperature going up to 25°C today – in May – how on earth am I going to cope in the summer with all the hot flushes? At least I will be able to use a deodorant again under my right arm! After today I only have three more sessions of radiotherapy to endure. One more week of treatment to go! I am so relieved; it is definitely dragging on now. I am so pleased we have holidays booked in June. I need them to look forward to and dream about, like yesterday when I was watching the common terns and dreaming about the arctic terns in the Shetlands.

Yesterday, I wore my bra all day and it didn't get too uncomfortable, but I was wearing the lightweight sponge prosthesis. I will do the same today. It doesn't look so good, which is a bit of a problem as I have to go to work and see patients. It is at the hospice, though, and they ought to understand. It makes for an entertaining conversation, anyway! The weighted silicon prosthesis was pressing too hard against my chest wall. It was making the whole area feel uncomfortably tight. The sponge is definitely better. If I can manage with this one it may mean I don't have to be a recluse next week and until the area settles down. I am wondering about going to the cinema or even the theatre next week. At least whilst sitting in the dark you can undo a bra if it is uncomfortable, provided you do it up again before the lights go back on! That is an advantage of the sponge prosthesis. As it is light it stays in place if the bra is undone. If I had the heavy one in place and had to undo the bra at the back, I would be sitting in the theatre with my left breast drooping a bit but my right breast sitting in my lap. Not so clever!

Friday 25 May

People are saying I am looking better and, yes, I am beginning to admit it myself. When I look back I now realise how ill I had become. I hope that is all now in the past. I want to continue to monitor my progress. I need to set myself realistic goals and work towards them.

When I am in the Shetlands I dream of revisiting Hermaness. That is a huge undertaking and will also depend on the weather. The walk is over peat bog, keeping a close lookout for dive-bombing bonxies (great skuas), to the cliff edge to view the deep blue sea between the island of Unst and Muckle Flugga and the neighbouring gannet colonies. The other reward is a fantastic view of puffins, razorbills and guillemots. If I get there at the end of June, in five weeks' time, I will know I have regained my strength. It will be an indication of not just physical wellbeing but mental and spiritual health as well.

The weather is cooler now and it's raining. Last night we spent time in the garden, it was so warm. I moved the guinea pig run and then started to clear the patio of strips of fencing. After hammering all the rusty nails flat to make the wood transportable, I took them to the skip this morning. I am thrilled. My arms feel a bit tired but the muscles don't hurt even after using a hammer for a couple of hours. This is great news!

Underneath the strips of wood I found an old skipping rope. A few years ago I could reach between eighty and a hundred without stopping or tripping up. I wondered if I would even be able to turn the rope, whether my arms would cope with the action. I then wondered if I could jump. Would I have enough strength in my legs? I turned the rope and jumped a couple of times but my co-ordination was poor. I tried again and got to three, and then I got to nine. This afternoon I managed seventeen and then thirty before having to stop to catch my breath. I am very pleased. This is an excellent way to get fit again, and hopefully even fitter than before. I am so glad I cleared the patio of junk! The only problem is that I spotted my reflection in the shed window as I skipped. My left breast was moving up and down rhythmically but the soft, lightweight sponge prosthesis wasn't moving. It looked so funny, I had to laugh.

Reflection: work and illness

'Everyone else is allowed time off for "a virus"; everyone else can be given a 'sick-note' for "back-pain" or "stress" but the doctor keeps going.'

That has always been my attitude to my work. Until November 2006 I had only ever had one or two days off sick in my entire working life. OK, I had had maternity leave and several years when I did very little work whilst the girls were young, but when I was meant to work, I worked. In the past I have been very critical of my younger colleagues who fail to live up to these strict standards. My father, a consultant dermatologist, demonstrated these standards (he needed to be admitted to hospital before he missed a clinic), and the same attitude was reinforced at medical school. After all, patients have booked appointments to see you, and you can't let them down. The fact that you were seeing them and managing them when you really wanted to be in bed, and concentration was poor, was irrelevant!

In spite of my attitude to work within the medical profession, reinforced by the comments of patients that doctors shouldn't be sick, I hope I have always been supportive of my patients' need to have time to recuperate. In fact, since suffering severe stress at work myself, but without taking any sick leave, I have been almost insistent that those in similar situations have time off work, to give them time to recover and reflect on their future.

Summer 2006

The weather was extremely hot in July 2006. My workload was too heavy. I was working two days a week in general practice, but up to nine surgeries a week if one of my partners was on holiday. I was also working at the hospice two mornings a week and on call once a week. As well as the regular daytime work, I was on call as a police surgeon for mid and south Bucks one night a week, or twenty-four hours over the weekend. Most weeks, I would have to drive the sixteen miles through the Chilterns at least once, during the night, down to High Wycombe after midnight. I used to enjoy seeing the badgers, foxes, deer and rabbits but I had reached fifty in May 2006 and I was beginning to question how much longer I could cope with the broken nights. My work and patients were beginning to suffer.

As well as my work, I was also trying to support my daughters by attending concerts and theatrical performances. In addition, I was working towards the diploma in the philosophy of medicine of the Society of Apothecaries. The written exam was in the middle of July.

The exam was in London. The weather was very hot and I had been badly bitten on my legs. By the end of the exam the whole of my right leg had swollen up. It seemed to be twice the size of the left. It was very uncomfortable! Although I had time off for the exam I had to work again the following day. I continued to work with very swollen legs, and by the following week I had developed cellulitis (infection under the surface of the skin), first around my right ankle and then around my left. In fact, I watched it bubbling up around my left ankle. It was quite alarming. I wondered if I would need intravenous antibiotics but it gradually resolved with oral medication.

I should have had time off work. I should have gone home and elevated my ankles. Instead, I was on call overnight for the police. At 2 a.m. I had to drive down to Wycombe. All I wanted to do was lie down but I felt obliged to go. My legs were throbbing, and it hurt to drive. When I arrived at the custody suite, the prisoner was reassured by the police officer guarding him that the doctor had been called to take blood from him, and nothing else. I found this quite a challenge. I was there to obtain a blood sample for the purposes of the Road Traffic Act, but to drive sixteen miles in the middle of the night, just to stick a needle in someone's arm, and then drive all the way back is not good use of my skills! The previous week in my philosophy and ethics exam I had written an essay on the place of Kantian, duty-based ethics in medicine. I argued that, as a forensic medical examiner, it is very important to remember Kant's philosophy to treat everyone as 'ends in themselves and not just means to an end'. We should respect everyone and not just 'use' them – especially prisoners. On that occasion I felt 'used' by the police and I felt the prisoner was being treated as a 'lesser mortal' who had to be processed, and not as a person in crisis. I consider it important to give the prisoner a chance to talk. Someone arrested for drink-driving has reached a crisis in his (or her) life. I try to listen and give them a chance to talk. That makes the sixteen-mile drive worthwhile. I drove *home that night, in pain, reflecting on whether I was getting too old for the job.*

I had never had such a major reaction to insect bites before, nor had I ever had cellulitis before. When I was diagnosed with breast cancer ten weeks later I wondered if there was a connection or whether it was just an unfortunate coincidence. I continued to work whilst suffering from cellulitis. It took a hospital admission for a mastectomy to make me slow down. It is so easy to believe you are indispensable, I'm not proud of it. It's time to give younger doctors a chance.

Saturday 26 May

We had a lovely pub lunch at the Rock of Gibraltar pub by the Oxford canal and then a super stroll along the canal looking and listening to the reed buntings and sedge warblers. We also saw a buzzard. On the way back we saw twelve red kites circling above the railway line at Bledlow. It was amazing to watch them all.

Bank holiday Monday 28 May

Today is a typical bank holiday Monday! Cold and pouring with rain!

I used this morning constructively; I sorted out my medical bags, in particular the out-of-date medication. This is a really good start. My bags need to be lighter so I can carry them into the custody suite or a patient's house. This seems to me to be a good indication I am nearly ready to go back to work; I'm planning in advance, not just existing!

I have been trying to decide all day whether I will go up to London tomorrow evening. Rachel is visiting Marian for half-term and they plan to queue up tomorrow morning, very early, for tickets for *The Lord of the Rings: the Musical*. I really want to see it. They will get tickets for the front row. If I don't go to London I won't see Rachel again until the end of June. I haven't seen her since Easter. The last time they invited me to join them I had to say no, because of the severe effects of chemo, and I couldn't travel up to Manchester to see Rachel playing in a musical, for the same reason.

I need to decide whether I am now well enough. I am working at the hospice in the morning and Veronica is taking me over to Oxford for my radiotherapy in the afternoon. I will feel tired after that but I can snooze on the train if necessary. Will my feet become too swollen for me to enjoy the theatre? But if we are on the front row there will be plenty of leg-room. I have to be well for Wednesday as I am on call all day for the police. However, I would really like to see Rachel. I want her to see me looking so much better. When I became ill I resolved that I wouldn't become so busy that I have to say, 'I can't see you, I'm working,' so I want to try. I will ask them to try to get me a ticket, and we will go from there.

Well, I guess that was a good bit of utilitarian decision-making, weighing up the pros and cons to maximise pleasure and minimise pain. I normally don't approve of hedonistic utilitarianism, feeling much more comfortable with Kantian duty-based ethics. But I did consider the maxim 'do unto others as you would have them do to you'. It is important that I am alert enough to work on Wednesday, but it is also important that I spend time with my daughters. What I am also learning is that I have a need for time to enjoy myself as well. I would love to see *The Lord of the Rings* anyway.

Wednesday 30 May

Well, I made it. It was touch and go, not because I was too tired, but because the radiotherapy department was so busy I was treated thirty minutes late. This meant I didn't get back to Aylesbury until 5 p.m. Fortunately, I managed to get a fast train from Princes Risborough so I could grab a bite to eat at Marylebone. Catching the tube was no problem. I managed the stairs with no difficulty. I also managed a brisk five-minute walk from Covent Garden to the theatre. Again, this was a good indication of my improvement as it was the theatre next to the Novello, so I know how many pauses I had needed on my way there before Easter. On that occasion it seemed such a long way to walk!

The special effects in *The Lord of the Rings* were amazing, I am so glad I went and it was great to see Rachel as well as Marian.

My chest wall is more uncomfortable, especially just under my arm. I spent most of yesterday afternoon and evening with my bra undone. It didn't look silly though; it was so cold and wet at the end of May, I went to London with a thick coat on. I don't remember the last time I wore a thick coat in London, it's been so mild.

I have had a very quiet day today but when it eventually stopped raining I tried skipping again. I skipped about hundred skips including sixty-six in a row!

Ethical reflection

I recently met a wonderful octogenarian. She was an in-patient. Normally, she lived on her own but with family support. She was a bit muddled initially, but just before her admission she had had the first cycle of chemotherapy. Her chemo regime was in tablet form and taken for two weeks at home, with a break before the next cycle. She was due to start the next cycle the following week. I decided to sit down with her and discuss this in detail.

She explained the detail of her regime. She said she had to take thirteen tablets in the morning; most were OK but she was struggling to swallow the big ones. I don't know which these were but I suspect they were the chemotherapeutic drugs, and the smaller ones the drugs to ward off the side-effects. She said she had coped with the effects but I wasn't so sure. She was trying to cope with chemotherapy at home, on her own. No wonder she was confused on admission.

I was really concerned. From my point of view, what was the point of her going through five more cycles? For her there was no chance of cure and no guarantee of improved quality of life after chemo. The one thing I was concerned about was significant morbidity whilst on the chemo; she might manage one more cycle but not five.

I didn't know how much she understood about her treatment, or what she hoped to achieve, so I decided to ask her what she thought the treatment was for. She seemed to think it was for her pain, but she made it clear that she was more than happy with the slow-release opiates we had sorted out for her. Once I had established that pain was her main problem, I discussed with her the fact that this could be managed by us by adjusting her pain relief, and that the chemo was to treat her disease. Suddenly, she looked relieved that she could choose not to take the medication provided her family were also happy.

Was it appropriate to reflect on my own experiences when talking to her?

Months ago, when I had been examining the use of casuistry in medical ethics following my dissertation, I wondered if I would become my own 'paradigm case', a case that would profoundly affect ethical decision-making, by learning from that experience. As doctors we all learn from the patients we meet and the better we listen, the more we learn. The conclusion of my dissertation was the importance of really listening to discern what the patient really needs, especially in palliative care. That's why it is so important to sit down and spend time with the patients at the hospice. Sometimes, listening takes a long time and requires a lot of patience. I had to go back to my patient and have another attempt to listen to her, once I had sorted out the facts from her medical notes, so that I could work out what she was trying to say. Listening in this case is a specialist skill.

By listening, I could tell she was struggling with the tablets and did not really have a good idea why she was on chemotherapy. I also managed to work out that her main problem was pain, and that was what she wanted help with. When she was admitted she was confused; this may have been due to her pain relief or her chemo or both. The confusion started to improve. This may be due to switching her to a different opiate or just giving her time and space to recover with good nursing care.

Once we had established that her pain could be easily managed with strong analgesia, the chemotherapy no longer seemed so important to her (she thanked me for clearing up a few points).

My own experience of chemotherapy does affect my thinking, but I think that I will use it appropriately to aid decision-making. I am now fifty-one and, prior to my chemotherapy, I was a little overweight but otherwise very healthy, only needing inhalers for very well-controlled asthma. This lady was wonderful, but she was already in her eighties and rather lonely, and so coming to the end of a long and fruitful life. For me, chemotherapy was part of a package of treatments with the potential to cure my breast cancer. I have plenty of family and the possibility of living into my eighties. This lady is already in her eighties and the chemotherapy was purely palliative. To endure six cycles of chemotherapy and then die anyway would be so sad for her and her family.

The four principles approach to biomedical ethics can be used to establish appropriate care here:
1. Respect for autonomy – freedom of choice – should be examined in the light of what the patient really wanted, which with careful listening was, in fact, better pain relief.
2. Beneficence – doing good; doing our best for the patient. This was achieved by giving her time, excellent nursing care, pain relief, and a visit from our hairdresser to name a few simple actions to restore her self-esteem.
3. Non-maleficence – not doing harm. We needed to question if offering this lady further chemotherapy would, in fact, cause more harm than good. In the end we all agreed it would.
4. Justice – fairness; appropriate use of resources. This lady's primary need was for good care and pain relief.

I know that, at the moment, if anyone offered me more chemo, I would refuse it; I've been through enough, but that is not the point. I will happily chat to patients about the risks and benefits of chemo, and all the problems that they face, in a balanced way, but I felt chemotherapy would cause more harm than good for this lady and that this was not a priority for her.

One final thought, and probably the important lesson to learn from this case, is that I could not have gone through the ordeal of chemotherapy without the support of my husband, daughters and friends cooking meals and just checking up on me. If I had been living on my own, without the reassuring sound of someone else around keeping an eye on me, I don't think I would have kept going. If I could not do that at the age of fifty, I certainly would not have managed at the age of eighty.

I saw the lady again a few days later. I hardly recognised her; she looked radiant and beautiful. She was relaxed, out of bed, chatting to the other patients. They had all had their hair done. She was ready to go home. For me this was clear evidence that we had all made the right decision.

June 2007

Friday 1 June
<u>Reflection on early retirement</u>

I spoke to the practice accountant yesterday. He gave me some information to mull over. He was talking about pensions. He knows I've been having treatment for cancer and assumed I would need to retire early on health grounds. When I first became ill I spoke with Nick about early retirement, say at fifty-five, to 'make the most of the time I have left'. We don't know if I am cured or not.

At present, I am sore where I am having radiotherapy but otherwise I feel so much better; my strength is returning and my enthusiasm for work increasing. However, I have learned so much through my illness and I have begun a theology course. I am thriving on the course's reflective and academic elements. I love medicine but there are other things I can do as well. Veronica, a retired teacher, has a great pastoral role among the elderly in church. I would love to be involved there. I was thinking about that earlier this week, and then remembered I was meant to be going back to work. That will have to wait. The question is – for how long? It would be very dishonest to say I can't work at all. After all, I have been working, doing hospice work and a little police work, but in these jobs you can set your own pace. General practice is different; you have to be able to run, both metaphorically and literally, to keep up. I won't be able to have a break if I am getting tired in the middle of a surgery. It is physically and mentally very demanding. I am due to go back to seeing patients in the practice at the beginning of July. I need to see how I get on.

At the moment, I think it is probably extremely reasonable to consider the possibility that, mentally and physically, my body will have had enough of the demands of general practice considerably before I am sixty. Until yesterday, I had no idea what retirement on grounds of 'ill health' meant. I need to see how I am when I go back.

These are my first thoughts on the subject. I think it is important to address it. It will be good to reread this and revisit the subject once I have returned to practice.

I am also aware that of all the work I do, the hospice work and possibly Mental Health Act assessments are the most rewarding. These are areas I may be able to focus on in the future, without the other pressures.

Saturday 2 June

Great day!

At 9.30 a.m. today I completed my radiotherapy! This is fantastic! It doesn't mean I'm fully recovered but at least all that treatment is over. I came home after we had been shopping in Aylesbury market and slept! I then cooked a celebratory lunch that we ate outside on the patio. At least this weekend is better than last.

Monday 4 June

'Cooked' – that's what my chest wall feels like: 'cooked'! It looks extremely red and is now feeling sore. The worst place is just under my arm. I think there are tiny little blisters developing there but at least it hasn't ulcerated.

Yesterday, when I weighed myself, my weight was lower than it had been since before Easter but today my ankles are very swollen again and my hands feel puffy. I expect I will need to wee more than once overnight. It will be interesting to see what my weight is in the morning. Tonight, I am five pounds heavier than I was yesterday and I was breathless again coming upstairs.

Will I ever get better?

This morning was OK; I managed 100 skips in a row! I also went for a lovely walk by the canal this afternoon listening to the willow warblers, chiffchaffs, sedge warblers and skylarks, in particular. The canal was green and yellow. There were yellow flags growing on the water's edge, masses of buttercups and some beautiful bright yellow water lilies in the canal as well.

I have spent this evening sorting out my accounts. June is always a busy month for administration with my accounts to do, and as I always have my GP annual appraisal in July, there is that to sort out too.

Reflections about work

Whilst sorting things out this evening I came across the General Medical Council's list of 'duties of a doctor'. I thought it was time to revisit some of these, as I am preparing to go back into general practice.

The first consideration is that doctors must 'make the care of patients their first concern'. What does this actually mean? I think, in many ways, I was in danger of taking this so literally that I failed to look after myself. Surely this is a serious issue in my profession. The doctor worries so much about the care of her patients that she neglects her own health and her family. Isn't that the lesson I am learning at the moment? There is a definite need for a proper balance. If you don't look after yourself the patients suffer in the long run. Patients want to see the doctor they are used to and they can't if she is off sick.

'Treat every patient politely and considerately', 'respect patients' dignity and privacy'. Yes, I believe I do.

'Listen to patients and respect their views.' That is what I keep teaching to the junior doctors at the hospice. It is so important to really listen; not to guess or assume you know what the patient wants, but to spend time working out what they really need. That was why I started doing my ward round carrying a chair around with me, rather than my stethoscope. It's funny to think I started wandering around the ward with a chair only a couple of months before I needed to sit down to talk to patients, because I couldn't stand up for very long, once I had started my chemo.

'Give patients information in a way they can understand', 'respect the right of patients to be fully involved in decisions about their care'. Those two go hand in hand. How can patients start to make a decision if they don't understand the options? However, as I made clear when I was diagnosed, the doctor requires wisdom to discern whether a normally competent patient is capable of a rational decision when in mental turmoil following a cancer diagnosis, or similar.

'Keep their professional knowledge and skills up to date.' That is what is worrying me. My last GP surgery was in November last year. I have been reading philosophy and theology and the newspaper but I *have spent very little time keeping up to date. I have maintained the skills needed for palliative care, but what about my consultation skills for general practice? I fear they will be rusty. I must try to update before returning, but there is little time, and I want to do other things.*

Wednesday 6 June

I have spent the day cleaning, dusting and throwing things away. I'm tired but at least I am managing to achieve more in a day now.

My chest wall is beetroot-coloured, I need to sort out the right dressings to keep it comfortable. It's getting much more difficult to get off to sleep. I'm getting pain in my left hip when I lie on my left side but it can be quite painful lying on my right side unless I get my arm in exactly the right position. I know it may deteriorate further for the next four or five days before things start to settle down.

Thursday 7 June

I had my theology tutorial today. We were talking about parables and miracles. Mike, the tutor, mentioned that in one of the other modules one of the challenges is to write a parable. I want to think about this and see what I can come up with.

During the tutorial my mobile rang, but I elected not to answer it; I shouldn't have had it on anyway. When I got home I listened to my voice message. It was Marian. She sounded really upset, begging me to answer. I phoned her straight back but there was no answer. I left a message for her but tried again later. Still no answer! I began to panic. What was wrong? I felt I had really let her down, not being there in her hour of need. My imagination ran wild; she lives and works in London, and it's not always a safe place. I realised I didn't have any other means of contacting her, nor did I have the phone number of her flatmate. I considered phoning her sister to see if she knew more, but I didn't want to get her into a panic too, and it might be confidential.

Eventually, Marian phoned back. She was so excited, she had been offered the lead in a good new musical and wanted to let me know. I'm really pleased, but told her that next time she leaves me a message, not to make it sound as if she has just been raped. Actors!

Friday 8 June

I'm beginning to peel under my arm, and it is increasingly tender under the elastic of my bra. It certainly burns at night.

This morning I switched to a new handbag. My old one was falling apart. It was time to empty it out and sort out what I really needed.

As I was removing everything I was reflecting on the scriptures 'come to me all who labour and are heavy laden, and I will give you rest', and 'my yoke is easy, my burden light' (Matt. 11:28, 30). I was aware my bag was far too heavy. Why else had it fallen apart so quickly? The bag and purse were full of unnecessary receipts, envelopes and other scraps of paper, but more significantly, in a handbag which I had bought at Wycombe General Hospital on the day I had my mastectomy, I found both a hairbrush and a comb. I didn't have sufficient hair to brush then and I still don't. I have been carrying them around everywhere but I have never used them!

Is there a parable here? We carry worries around with us. There is no rest while we worry. I was carrying rubbish and unnecessary items around with me, weighing me down, in the same way we carry around unnecessary worries that Jesus asks us to give to him.

I spent the day getting the house and garden ready for us to go on holiday. The lawn is more like a meadow but it's great for the guinea pigs. Marian phoned whilst I was cooking tea and moving the guinea pig run. Nick said she sounded furtive. She wanted to talk to me. I tried ringing her back, but her phone went straight to voicemail. She was on a train. Marian always rings us when she's on a train and Rachel when she's about to get on a bus!

What could be going on this time? She obviously didn't want to tell her dad.

I was struggling; I needed to get the chicken wire run moved but every time I was interrupted I needed to stand up again. I was kneeling down in the garden. It is hard to get down and get up again. I need to really pull myself up with my arms. It is difficult in the garden without furniture, or stairs, or cupboards to hold onto.

I eventually got back to Marian. She didn't know how to break the news to me. She said she had met a 'lovely' lady today when she was rehearsing the play she is in. They were rehearsing at a pub in Islington, the venue for the performances. She explained that there is a play being performed at present and one of the actors was there. She looked straight at Marian and said 'Don't I know you from somewhere?' Marian said that she certainly did and said she was 'Marian Elizabeth… Marian Elizabeth *Butland*.' Marian had instantly recognised the other actor as Mrs C! (not her stage name). They talked! I am so impressed with Marian; it must have been quite a shock. She last spoke to her more than a decade ago, but I only recently showed Marian my write-up of what really happened, and I am so glad I did. This actor was the woman who shouted at me between consultations, mocked me and threw things at me whilst she was my practice manager. The woman who wrote of me that I was the 'nastiest, most vindictive and wicked person to ever walk this earth' and sent it to the BMA. Among other things she told Marian that she is a grandma and that her husband (and my former GP partner) would be picking her up. I'm so glad she didn't suggest Marian say 'Hi!' to him.

I thought this might happen at some time. We knew she had been through drama school once her husband left the practice, and that she had performed at that venue before, and Marian often performs there. I am very proud of Marian; she clearly behaved so well towards her, and showed her respect.

Saturday 9 June

Off to Devon today.

I struggled to get off to sleep last night. I was uncomfortable and hot but I also kept worrying about Marian's meeting with Mrs C.

Reflection

I wonder how I would have coped if this had happened whilst I was having chemotherapy? I am certainly glad that it happened when I completed my treatment, but it has stirred up some difficult memories again. Marian said Mrs C didn't look at her again, and didn't say anything to her when she left. I wonder what she was thinking. At least she didn't just spit at my daughter, or turn her back on her when she realised who she was. In the past she had no idea how to treat people or behave; could that have changed?

I recalled last night that when I talked to her youngest son (aged eighteen at the time) two years after I left the surgery, he too was very polite and chatted to me naturally. However, the following week Mrs C had descended on me with another lad playing the role of the 'heavy'; in front of several people who knew her, she had, almost incoherently, ranted that I would be beaten up if I ever talked to one of her sons again. I'm not planning to do that!

It probably is a good thing, though, that we were about to go on holiday, and had already booked tickets for An Inspector Calls in Torquay this evening, otherwise I would have been so tempted to go and see the play she is in. I have resisted that temptation for years, but I usually have no information about what she is in. The performance area at that theatre is so intimate that she would be well aware of my presence in the audience (if she recognised me with very short hair). The temptation is to find out how she would cope. Is she a good enough actor to mask her feelings completely? It will probably happen at some time. I'm not perfect but I have resisted the temptation until now!

People have asked me why I didn't involve the police when I left the practice. It was difficult as Dr C was a respected police surgeon, but after the incident in public involving her son, I did seek the help of the police. An officer visited her at the surgery and simply warned her about her behaviour, which was enough.

Sunday 10 June – Kingsteignton

The weather was wonderful today. As thunderstorms are forecast for tomorrow, it was the day to go up on Dartmoor. It was amazing. The ground underfoot is so like the Shetlands, and the trees as few. The skylarks were singing beautifully and the pipits parachuting to the ground. We could hear a snipe calling. I managed to walk for three and a half hours over rough terrain and peat bog. I fell over twice in the long grass (but Nick fell once!) My balance isn't perfect and I should have had a stick with me. Crossing streams on stones and climbing up and down over stones wasn't easy, but I made it! I was exhausted at the end of the walk, but we had a proper cream tea at Princetown.

I managed to get the treated area of my chest wall comfortable for our walk today but it was getting sore in the car on the way back. Last night, it was so sore I wanted to cry. It is hard to believe it could get any redder. At least I only have two more days until I reach the tenth day after my last dose of radiotherapy. I hope it is true that it will start to settle after that. I would like to go swimming in the hotel pool before we leave. We'll see.

Monday 11 June

The skin under my arm is no longer sore so I decided to see if I could tolerate deodorant again. Admittedly, since I have had radiotherapy, I don't sweat so much under my right arm, but it has been a problem trying to keep fresh without using deodorant. I am pleased to say it didn't sting. I feel so much more confident wearing deodorant under both arms! I don't have to carry baby wipes around all the time.

I realised I wouldn't be able to go for a swim unless we bought some safety pins. We managed to get some so I plucked up courage to pin the sponge prosthesis into my swimming costume. I was concerned that the red area on my chest wall would alarm the other bathers, but it was mostly covered; it didn't look as bad as I had feared. Amazingly, it didn't sting when I immersed myself in the pool. My swimming stroke was very weak but at least I managed to swim. I didn't spend long in the pool but it was a good start.

Wednesday 13 June

I am trying very hard to eat enough fruit and vegetables and get enough exercise.

At last, I have seen some research that is helpful to me. In Saturday's Independent *there was a report of some research that I must look up when I get home. It reported research on women followed up after a diagnosis of early breast cancer. That's the point, it's sensible advice about what to do now, rather than what I should have done! Not how to prevent the disease but how to stay well. It is, in fact, very timely advice! The research seems to suggest that eating the recommended five portions of fruit and vegetables a day, plus thirty minutes of brisk walking per day (six out of seven days a week) halved the risk of recurrence in the women followed up. However, the women needed to adopt both these healthy lifestyles, not just one or the other, to have any effect.*

I need to look at the original article but at least there is nothing wacky or difficult about the advice. It's not as if I am being advised to start having daily enemas or switch to a vegetarian diet. This is just excellent advice for anyone and I love fruit and vegetables anyway!

It will require some discipline to keep up the exercise and ensure I always have enough fruit and vegetables in the house. I am sure I have been eating well enough recently, but of course the exercise is another matter. I am only now well enough to undertake 'brisk' walking!

I wonder if it will be extrapolated to 'prevention'. At least I know my daughters already live that sort of healthy lifestyle.

Lifestyle advice is difficult. After all since, I was diagnosed with breast cancer, research has been published indicating that daily consumption of small amounts of alcohol can accelerate the development of breast cancer. Well, I was drinking alcohol most days – but not when on call for the police – but only at the level that was 'good for my heart'. I am certainly not going to stop drinking alcohol; it's a matter of quality of life. What is the point of cutting out things I enjoy in moderation just, possibly, to prolong my life by a year or two?

(On reading the original article I note that ladies were only recruited for the trial after they had been diagnosed for two years. This, of course, eliminated anyone who developed early recurrence and ensured participants could undertake brisk walking.)

Thursday 14 June

Yesterday was a long but lovely day, catching up with relatives and friends. We met Nick's nieces Fran and her younger half-sisters Maria and Paula. I hadn't seen Maria and Paula since before their mother died; they now both have babies of their own. It was interesting talking to Maria and Paula. Maria was fourteen and Paula twelve when their mother developed abdominal swelling and was diagnosed with advanced cancer. Our daughters were very young at the time and it wasn't long after the death of Nick's dad, their grandfather. Maria and Paula said they didn't realise how ill their mother was; they thought she was going to get better, and none of them believed their mother felt she knew she was terminally ill. How sad it must have been so hard for all of them. It is lovely to see how close the three of them are.

We had a lovely walk, in glorious weather, at Lizard Point. Unfortunately, the chough family had fledged, so we didn't see that stunning rare crow, but, at least I managed to walk really comfortably and freely along the narrow paths.

It was great to visit our friends Phil and Caroline Rodda and their family in Scorrier (in Cornwall) during the evening. We visited them just after I was diagnosed, so it was great to see them again at the end of my treatment, and to be given plenty of their Cornish cream!

Yesterday was great but today I am very sore. I have struggled to make my dressings comfortable. I have run out of mepilex; fortunately the local Boots has some. It is not cheap to buy, but worth it.

It poured with rain last night. We ended up eating Cornish pasties looking at a small wood called 'Butland Plantation'. At the edge of the plantation I spotted a hazel bush and I was impressed to see there were some well-formed hazelnuts. I now have a photo of hazelnuts in Butland Plantation!

We went round Drogo Castle in the afternoon. I struggled up and down the stairs – there were often no handrails to hold on to. Not ideal for the disabled!

I improved when we reached Exeter. We went to Exeter Cathedral. It was good to go to evensong.

Saturday 16 June

What a difference having the right dressing makes. The mepilex dressing is so comfortable even though the irradiated area is red and peeling badly. I am determined to wear my proper prosthesis for our family party in two days time.

I was tired after walking around Saltram House. I am worried about whether I will cope back at the surgery in just over two weeks' time. Sitting down and standing up are still difficult, and kneeling down on the floor and picking things up is a real problem. I don't know how long this sort of thing takes to clear up.

Am I going back to work too soon? I've got to try.

This afternoon we went for a lovely walk in the pouring rain at Plymbridge to see a family of peregrine falcons. We saw one adult and two fledglings. It was wonderful how much more energy I had after lunch and a short rest!

I think Nick is more relaxed about my illness now. When it was pouring with rain I wondered where to put my camera to stop it getting wet. He suggested taking out my sponge prosthesis and putting the camera in there instead.

Sunday 17 June

Hot flushes are becoming a major problem at night. Nick is fast asleep with pyjama trousers on and a thick duvet over him and I have had to get up to cool off. I was so sweaty, in spite of sleeping without the duvet over me and removing my top. I know some women say they even have to change the sheets. That must be awful! How can you go on holiday, or stay overnight in a hotel if you need to change the sheets during the night?

It has been really good to have the occasional bath whilst we have been away. Of course we have a bath at home but in December 2005 we had a new bathroom suite fitted with a large shower/bath. Apart from the fact it takes a lot of water to fill, so I feel at times it is a waste of water, we also had handrails removed when the wall was retiled. They had been fitted by the previous occupants, one of whom was disabled. The bath in our accommodation has handles on both sides, and a handrail on the wall. It was so good to feel secure getting into and out of the bath, even when not wearing my glasses. Of course, being able to see adequately is important too. I hadn't realised how important sight was for good balance until now. I'm not too bad balancing on my right leg but much worse on my left. I can understand why my father, with Parkinson's disease, fell over and fractured ribs when he was unable to wear his glasses. His balance was already compromised and then he also could not see properly.

Monday 25 June

Nick drove me to Stansted Airport. Amazingly I landed at Sumburgh on time. This is the end of June but I needed my woollen hat and gloves, and my thick coat when I got off the plane in the Shetlands, but, at least it wasn't raining. It had been raining in London when we left, and pretty cold there too!

I picked up my hire car and immediately drove to the lighthouse at Sumburgh Head. The last time we had been there in June last year, the visibility had been so poor we couldn't see the sea. This time I could. I could see, and photograph, the guillemots on the rocks and a solitary seal below. But the puffins came to me. They are wonderful birds popping in and out of their burrows just the other side of the wall. They are impossible to miss and such fun to watch!

After my puffin 'fix' I drove the length of Mainland in just under an hour to Toft and the ferry terminal. The roads are fantastic with so little traffic, but I was aware that I hadn't driven so far since I was first ill. The short ferry journey was smooth between Mainland and Yell. It was good to have a few minutes on Yell to buy some wine for my hosts, Peter and Janet and the best thick locally made oatcakes and some Orkney cheddar for me! I then drove across Yell to catch the 4 p.m. ferry to Fetlar.

What a joy to arrive on Fetlar, to be greeted by the curlews and oyster catchers. The drive over to Peter and Janet's is so beautiful.

They have such a lovely house close to a freshwater loch (Papil Water), adjacent to a sand spit separating the loch from the sea. Tresta is a wonderful beach! It was so good to see Peter and Janet again and then to go for a walk down to the beach before supper. As usual the great skuas (bonxies) were enjoying their beach party at the edge of the loch whilst ringed plovers were running around on the grass.

Wednesday 27 June

It was quite windy yesterday and cold but I managed to sort out the difference between a whimbrel and a curlew. This is the birdwatcher's equivalent of 'sorting out the sheep from the goats', bearing in mind that in the Middle East sheep and goats can look quite similar.

The weather was very misty this morning, but I decided to visit Unst anyway. I love Unst, the most northerly of the Shetland Isles. I practised walking with my stick over quite rough ground. It was very successful; I managed quite a distance. If the weather improves I will come back to Unst at the end of the week to walk round Hermaness nature reserve – the most northerly point on the island.

Thursday 28 June

Blue sky, warm sunshine, blue sea; the world looks so amazing! I had a wonderful walk over a headland along the coast of Fetlar. There are new stiles which mark the route, but I struggled to get over them. They seem to have been designed for people with very long legs!

I have now discovered two more functions for my walking stick. You can stick it in the ground in front of you to see if the peat bog is firm enough to hold your weight, and you can hold it above your head to ward off the dive bombing bonxies. It is certainly a very useful walking aid!

Friday 29 June

Well I made it! I had set myself a goal some weeks ago of walking to the cliff tops looking out towards Muckle Flugga lighthouse, and the gannet colonies, from Hermaness, and I made it. OK, I didn't walk quite as far as last year and the ground was less boggy and it wasn't so windy, but I made it. The great bonus was that because the weather was wonderful – sunny and calm – I could sit near the edge of the cliff among the puffins. I sat and read and rested whilst the puffins walked to and fro in and out of their burrows, or greeted their mates by banging their beaks.

Reflection on goals

It was a wonderful target to have set myself and a great feeling to have achieved my goal. After all, at Easter I could just about walk 400 yards on the flat and really struggled to climb stairs, but today I walked two miles uphill over peat bog and two miles back. It took me just over fifty minutes to reach the cliff edge, but I spent at least two hours enjoying the view, the birds and the atmosphere before going back. I think it was then reasonable to celebrate with a half of the locally brewed stout in the newly opened bar nearby!

I only really have one more target to achieve and that is getting back to general practice next week. I am getting quite anxious about it. I feel so out of touch. Will I cope? Will I be too tired? Will my ankles swell up too much and become too uncomfortable? I hope I can meet everyone's expectations of me. I think it will be hard.

July 2007

Tuesday 3rd July

Oh dear! When I woke up yesterday morning and looked out of the window over the bay I knew we were in trouble. It was foggy, even though it had been really windy during the night. I drove back to Sumburgh airport as planned but knew I was in for a long day. The ninety-minute flight back to Stansted was cancelled and we were put on the overnight ferry to Aberdeen.

There are some advantages to being a cancer patient: at least I had some anti-emetics with me. It was a bit rough to start with but at least I enjoyed my free supper!

Even so, yesterday was an ordeal and a reminder that I am not completely well. Initially, I wasn't allocated a cabin, or even a reclining chair. When I thought I was going to have to spend the whole night sitting in a chair I wanted to cry. I wouldn't have coped; my ankles would have been so swollen, and after a night sitting in a chair I would still have a flight, and several train journeys ahead! I approached the reception desk on board and explained my problem, saying I was a 'cancer patient', and I was put on a waiting list for a bed. They found me one. They said it was the last one left, sharing with three others, but I didn't mind. I even ended up on the lower bunk, thanks to the generosity of one of the other ladies. I think I would have struggled in and out of the top bunk, even though it was reasonably calm! Walking up and downstairs on board was bad enough. My balance is still not wonderful!

I discovered the trials of travelling on my own. At least I didn't have a five-year-old child with me as well, like one other passenger. The terrorism alert level was at 'severe' after the failed car bomb at Glasgow airport at the weekend. I couldn't leave my luggage safely anywhere. I couldn't ask anyone to watch it whilst I went to the loo; it was very hard. We had checked our luggage in at Sumburgh, so when they announced our flight was cancelled, the luggage was returned to us on the conveyor belt, but they forgot to announce that. The first most people knew about it was hearing a very anxious announcement that, unless passengers removed their luggage immediately, it would be removed by security. At the same time we were watching the news reports about the flaming jeep crashing into Glasgow airport terminal.

Anyway I eventually got home at 1 p.m. today, almost twenty-four hours later than planned. I should have been working at the hospice this morning. It seems terribly irresponsible to fail to get back from a holiday in time to go back to work, especially as I didn't even travel abroad. That's the Shetlands for you. Our junior doctor advised me to go to Thailand next time!

Friday 6 July

I have now completed two days back at the surgery, seeing patients. I worked Wednesday afternoon and Thursday morning. I slept most of Thursday afternoon. There was a wonderful flower arrangement in my room from everyone at the surgery, to greet my return. You could smell the fragrance of the lilies in reception!

I'm glad I'm back, but it wasn't easy. I was really nervous. Would my consultation skills still be adequate? I also felt so out of date and wondered how much I had forgotten. In the end Rachel, my practice manager, and my receptionists were so helpful and so encouraging I needn't have worried. My ankles were swollen and I was walking rather slowly at the end of each surgery. I certainly couldn't have dashed off to an emergency, but I coped. I know some of the patients gained from the time I gave them.

Before my first surgery I put a notice up in the waiting room:

A message from Dr Hazel Butland

Thank you so much for all your support, gifts and good wishes during my illness.

I am feeling much better but still recovering from some of the effects of the treatment.

I have not found it easy being a patient but I hope I have learnt from the experience!

Epilogue

November 2007

I am so slow to learn! I have just been rereading my journal. I was anxious about returning to general practice in July, but I thought I would cope. After all, I was only going to be doing two surgeries a week. Obviously, I would still be working at the hospice and doing some daytime police work but it was still much less than I had been doing.

I had been right to be worried. I tried to keep going but at the beginning of September I realised I had to give up the police work. My arms ached after I had been driving a few miles. I couldn't keep driving to and from Wycombe. A twelve-hour shift, even in the daytime, was far too long. I wasn't safe driving by the end of the shift; I was desperate for sleep. I was physically and mentally exhausted, but we were going to have a holiday at the end of September. I thought things would improve after that.

The holiday was really special. We hired a narrow boat and spent a week relaxing and slowly cruising along the Grand Union Canal. Although I have spent many hours walking and reflecting beside the canal, neither of us had ever been on a narrow boat before. It was amazing. Steering was a challenge I had to master very quickly, and the locks were hard work. The long tunnels gave me time to think. As I steered into the tunnel it was just possible to see light at the other end.

I was relaxed and coped well with a limited amount of physical work but I overdid it one day and the next I struggled to walk any distance at all. I had to go back to bed.

I felt refreshed after the holiday and went back to work. I worked for another week before I was forced to acknowledge I wasn't coping. I had tried and tried and I had failed. It was too much.

I finally came to my senses on 2 October.

I had spent the morning working at the hospice. After lunch, I was involved in a training session for the nurses in day hospice. It was a role-play of a combined assessment of a new patient conducted by both a doctor and a nurse. Helen, the consultant, played herself; Jane, the nurse in charge, played herself, and I was the patient. I wasn't meant to be playing myself; I pretended I had cancer of the bowel and major social problems with my daughter's boyfriend.

They ushered me into the room and made me comfortable with extra pillows. The role-play went well, and I was enjoying myself, until Jane asked me if I had claimed all of the benefits I was entitled to. All of a sudden I found myself saying how exhausting it was filling in all the forms. I started to cry. This wasn't role-play any longer; this was me expressing real frustrations!

At the end of the role-play everyone was discussing the assessment and what they had gained from it, but I was so comfortable, I fell asleep.

It was time for reappraisal, to reduce my workload further, and to be referred to see a clinical psychologist

General practice is very hard work even for the young and able-bodied. I was working and sleeping and working and sleeping. My arms were painful and very weak. I went to occupational health and then confessed to Andy, my GP, that I needed to be signed off sick again. I had been so busy trying to work I hadn't noticed how weak and stiff my arms had grown again. I only knew they started to ache as soon as I tried to drive anywhere. I was far too tired to contemplate any exercise whilst I had been working at the surgery; I needed to conserve all my energy to concentrate on the patients, and make it to the end of the surgery. I even had a nap before afternoon surgery.

I knew I would be tired when I returned to work, but I thought it would slowly improve. Instead it got worse and worse. It was several weeks before I realised how much it would affect me psychologically and emotionally as well. Seeing other ladies with breast cancer started to effect me badly. I had another terrifying nightmare.

As soon as I was granted further sick leave I commenced hydrotherapy and a home exercise programme for my arms. It was amazing how quickly the pain in my arms resolved and I could stop painkillers. It has been a full-time job trying to get myself well again. I realised I was missing my walks – my times of quiet reflection as well as good exercise.

I now plan to focus on just one of my jobs. I hope to be able to continue to work at the hospice where I feel my experience both as a doctor and a patient is valued and most useful. By just working two mornings a week I really should have time for myself, time for my family and friends, and above all time to pray and reflect.

As I am writing this, I am again thinking about the long canal tunnels. As we entered the tunnel, it was just possible to see the light at the other end. It seemed to take such a long time to get there; I just had to keep going, focusing on the goal, the light, the end of the tunnel. It took so long to travel through the tunnels that, on one occasion, it was bright sunshine on entering but a torrential hailstorm when we emerged. That was Nick's turn to steer!

When I was first told I had cancer, I stood beside a stretch of the Grand Union Canal and reflected on the journey ahead. I knew it wouldn't be easy, but it was a path I had to follow. I spent many hours beside the canal but this was a new experience: deep inside a hill, travelling along the canal. Yes, there was light at the end of the tunnel, but like the change in the weather we experienced on emerging, I am a different person; I have changed. I have emerged from the end of the tunnel but I need a fresh start and new goals to focus on, realistic goals that are achievable but not so physically demanding.

I have just remembered the dream Sally at my surgery told me she had had, and that I recorded on 21 November, just before I had my mastectomy. She dreamt she was escorted around an insect house. I started as a larva and emerged as a butterfly. I think that is what I am trying to say: like a butterfly emerges from the chrysalis and is different from the larva and can't become a larva again, I have been on a long journey and I have learnt a great deal, but I am different now. I can't go back to how I was.

A friend, who has also had cancer, has wisely advised me to look at my working life before my diagnosis as 'completed', and not 'given up' because I failed.

This is the beginning of the next stage of my life.

Printed in the United Kingdom
by Lightning Source UK Ltd.
131505UK00001B/175-321/P